MW01182230

Keto Diet After 50

The Complete Ketogenic diet Guide For Man and Woman Over 50 with Easy Recipes & Meal Plan.

Including a Cookbook with Mouthwatering Recipes to Accelerate Weight Loss.

| Including a 30-Day Meal Plan |

Legal & Disclaimer

The information contained in this book and its contents is not designed to replace or take the place of any form of medical or professional advice; and is not meant to replace the need for independent medical, financial, legal or other professional advice or services, as may be required. The content and information in this book have been provided for educational and entertainment purposes only.

The content and information contained in this book has been compiled from sources deemed reliable, and it is accurate to the best of the Author's knowledge, information and belief. However, the Author cannot guarantee its accuracy and validity and cannot be held liable for any errors and/or omissions. Further, changes are periodically made to this book as and when needed. Where appropriate and/or necessary, you must consult a professional (including but not limited to your doctor, attorney, financial advisor or such other professional advisor) before using any of the suggested remedies, techniques, or information in this book.

Upon using the contents and information contained in this book, you agree to hold harmless the Author from and against any damages, costs, and expenses, including any legal fees potentially resulting from the application of any of the information provided by this book. This disclaimer applies to any loss, damages or injury caused by the use and application, whether directly or indirectly, of any advice or information presented, whether for breach of contract, tort, negligence, personal injury, criminal intent, or under any other cause of action.

You agree to accept all risks of using the information presented inside this book.

You agree that by continuing to read this book, where appropriate and/or necessary, you shall consult a professional (including but not limited to your doctor, attorney, or financial advisor or such other advisor as needed) before using any of the suggested remedies, techniques, or information in this book.

INTRODUCTION

Many may lack experience with a ketogenic diet. Here we look at the basic ideas and requirements regulating a ketogenic diet, which may be beneficial.

A ketogenic diet is basically any diet that allows the liver to shape ketone bodies, altering a person's metabolism to use fat instead of glucose. More precisely, a diet that restricts the intake of carbohydrates to a certain amount (usually below 100 grams per day) can be considered ketogenic, launching a series of devices. Protein and fat intake differ from weight loss targets. In the end, the determining factor of whether or not a diet is ketogenic is the presence (or absence) of carbohydrates.

Fuel metabolism and a ketogenic diet.

The body works on a mixture of carbohydrates, proteins, and fats, under "natural" conditions. As carbohydrates are eliminated from the diet small reserves of the body are rapidly exhausted. The body is being pushed to look for an alternative fuel source. One is the free fatty acids (FFA), which most body tissues can use. Not all organs should use FFA, however. The brain and nervous system, for example, cannot use FFA as a fuel; however, ketone bodies can be used.

Ketone bodies are a by-product of FFA separation in the liver. These do not function as a carbohydrate but as a fat source of fuel to tissues like the brain. If ketone bodies are formed at an accelerated rate, they build up in the blood causing a metabolic state called ketosis to develop. At the same time, glucose intake and development are increasing. Along with this, the protein degradation for use as an energy source is rising, which is also called "protein retention." Most people are attracted to the ketogenic diet because they are able to burn fat while retaining muscle mass.

Hormones and the ketogenic diet.

The changes mentioned above are triggered by ketogenic diets, mainly because of the effect on the two hormone levels: insulin and glucagon. Insulin is a "conservation hormone" responsible for passing nutrients from the blood to the tissues of the body. Therefore, the insulin allows glucose to accumulate in the muscles in the form of glycogen, and FFAs are contained in triglycerides in adipose tissue. Glucagon is a fuel-mobilizing hormone that activates the use of stores of glycogen, primarily contained in the liver, to provide the body with glucose.

When the diet eliminates carbohydrates, insulin levels decrease, and glucagon levels increase. It leads to increased FFA release from adipose tissue, and rapid FFA burning in the liver. What eventually contributes to the development of ketone bodies and the formation of a metabolic state called KETOS is the rapid burning of FFA in the Liver. In addition to insulin and glucagon, 11 other hormones are also affected, which helps to turn the body to fat instead of carbohydrates as a source of fuel in the compartment.

Exercise and a ketogenic diet

As with any other diet designed to burn fat, exercise will improve the ketogenic diet's efficacy. Nevertheless, a carbohydrate-free diet renders the exercise of high intensity difficult, whereas workouts of low intensity can be carried out. For this purpose, athletes wishing to conduct high-intensity workouts must include carbohydrates without affecting the ketosis impact.

CHAPTER ONE

What Is Ketogenic Diet

The history of this method began in the 1920s as an alternative to successfully treating epilepsy patients.

However, the diet became popular in the 1970s when the son of a very famous American producer used the ketogenic diet and managed to control the problem. He suffered about 5 seizures a day, and after starting the diet, he had none.

As early as the 1980s, an American doctor treated her husband, who had Alzheimer's disease at an advanced stage with the ketogenic diet. It used the inclusion of medium-chain triglycerides as well as those present in coconut oil.

What exactly is the ketogenic diet

The strategy present in the diet is an alternative rearrangement among the macronutrients that should make up the diet. Here the great source of energy becomes fat.

Did you know that consuming fat can be good for your body?

Protein remains consumed in adequate amounts and carbohydrates in minimal amounts. The physiological process of the human body is to break down fat into fatty acids and ketone bodies to get enough energy for cellular processes.

Without carbohydrates, the body is practically forced to break down beyond the fat that comes from food, which is already accumulated, fat usually accumulates due to excess carbohydrates in the diet, and this whole process leads to losing weight.

The evolution of the low-carb diet

In the low-carb diet, carbohydrate consumption is reduced. Thus, by eating more protein and fat, it is possible to increase the feeling of satiety, which leads directly to healthy weight loss.

I consider the ketogenic diet an evolution of the low-carb diet. The ketogenic diet is to reduce the amount of carbohydrate ingested drastically.

The principle assumes that decreasing carbohydrate consumption also lowers insulin stimulation. It ultimately improves the insulin profile, increasing its resistance, and decreasing the chances of developing various diseases such as diabetes, atherosclerosis, and even cardiovascular disease.

In the ketogenic diet, carbohydrate consumption is even lower, so the benefits are enhanced. In it, the recommended carbohydrate consumption is limited to a maximum of 50g per day.

CHAPTER TWO

The ketogenic diet for after 50

Over recent years, the keto diet has gained in popularity and has become a dietary program preferred by people of all ages. That said, this dietary roadmap could precipitate particularly significant health benefits for individuals over 50 years of age.

Keto Diet Summary

Scientifically called a ketogenic diet; this dietary program stressed the reduced consumption of carbohydrate-containing foods and increased fat intake. The decreased carbohydrate consumption is said to gradually put the participating dieters ' bodies in a biological and metabolic process known as ketosis.

Once ketosis is created, the body is particularly efficient in burning fat and converting these substances into energy by medical researchers. In addition, during this cycle, the body is assumed to metabolize fat into chemicals known as ketones, which are also said to provide substantial sources of energy.

[An accelerator is an intermittent fasting strategy that allows the body to reach the next available energy source or ketones that are extracted from stored fat by limiting carbs. In this lack of glucose, the body now burns fat for energy.]

There are a number of other specific ketogenic diets including:

- Targeted (TKD) those participating in this variant are gradually adding small amounts of carbohydrates to their diets.
- Cyclical (CKD) Adherents to this diet plan cyclically eat carbohydrates as every few days or weeks.

- High-protein Diet participants eat higher amounts of protein as part of their diet plans.

- Standard (SKD) Generally, this most widely used form of dietary intake significantly reduced carbohydrate concentrations (maybe as little as 5% of all dietary intake), along with protein-laden foods and a high amount of fat items (in some cases as much as 75% of all dietary requirements).

Keto Diet Benefits To Individuals Over 50

Adherents of the Keto diet, especially those aged 50 and older, are said to enjoy various potential health benefits including:

Increased physical and mental energy. For a variety of biological and environmental reasons, energy levels that drop as people grow older. Adherents of the Keto diet also experience an increase of strength and vitality. One explanation said phenomenon happens is because the body burns excess fat, which is synthesized into energy in turn. Additionally, systemic ketone synthesis tends to increase brain power and to enhance cognitive functions such as concentration and memory.

Improved Sleep. When individuals age, they tend to sleep less. Keto dieters often benefit more from exercise programs and become harder to tire. This occurrence may precipitate lengthier and more productive rest periods.

Metabolism. Aging people often experience a slower metabolism than they did in their younger days. Long-term keto dieters are experiencing better blood sugar control, which can improve their metabolic rates.

Weight Loss. Faster and more effective fat metabolism helps the body remove accumulated body fat, which may precipitate excess pound shedding. Furthermore, adherents are also thought to have a reduced appetite, which may lead to reduced caloric intake. Keeping off the weight is especially important when adults age when they may need fewer calories per day compared to living in the 20s or even 30s. Yet it is still necessary for older adults to get nutrient-rich food from this diet. Since it is normal for aging adults to lose muscle and energy, a nutritionist may prescribe a high protein-specific ketogenic diet.

Protection against Specific Illnesses. The risk of developing illnesses such as diabetes, mental disorders such as Alzheimer's, various cardiovascular diseases, different types of cancer, Parkinson's disease, Non-Alcoholic Fatty Liver Disease (NAFLD), and multiple sclerosis could be minimized by keto dieters over 50s.

Aging. Others find aging the most important risk factor for illness or disease in humans. Reducing aging is, therefore, the logical step towards reducing these disease risk factors.

Good news from the technical description of the ketosis cycle mentioned earlier shows the increased energy of the youth as a result, and because of the use of fat as a source of fuel, the body can go through a process where signals can be misinterpreted so that the mTOR signal is blocked and a lack of glucose is apparent where aging is stated to be slowed down.

Multiple studies have commonly recognized for years that caloric restriction can help slow aging and even increase lifespan. With the ketogenic diet, it is possible to have an effect on anti-aging without reducing the calories. The extended form of fasting used with a keto diet can also influence vascular aging.

CHAPTER THREE

How to Start a Keto Diet When You're Over 50?

As with any new diet or exercise plan, consulting your doctor before you start is always a good idea. Be mindful that outcomes differ between individuals. Once you've decided that the keto diet is right for you, removing all processed foods from your diet will be your first step.

Choosing a keto diet involves simplifying the food you eat and its ingredients. The food processed contains "any product that has been altered before consumption in some way." For example, any food that's processed, fried, bottled, frozen, or "fortified." That is to say goodbye to potato chips, crackers, sweet snacks, processed oils, items of imitation, "hot" and fast foods. Therefore you will also only need to buy high-quality meats, no more chicken or beef from intensive breeding.

You will find that shopping is simpler and cooking is easier once you get used to the fact that your meals are made up of whole foods. You're not going to consume less food, and you're going to consume the healthier food in its natural state. The aim of the keto diet is not to restrict calorie intake. In fact, you'll probably consume more calories than you're used to. But in the form of fats, those will be

For people over 50, you will enjoy a delicious steak, asparagus and zucchini sautéed in coconut oil and a bok choy (Chinese cabbage) and bacon salad while dinner consisted of lasagna with layers of refined pasta, high sugar tomato sauce, and a small amount of meat. Cow, pork, beef, bacon, potatoes, nuts, a range of cheeses, and rich leafy greens will be part of your meal. Low-fat diets are formerly a thing. Your body needs burning fat so you lose fat!

How to start a keto diet - step by step instructions

1. Reduce carbohydrate consumption.

Everything will work without it, the principal obvious move. To continue with up to 20 grams of carbohydrate per day, we reduce the intake. It allows the body to build all reserves of glucose and continue the transition to the energy production of fat.

2. Stir in the diet with coconut oil.

This contains MCT (medium-chain triglycerides), which are absorbed very quickly by the body and converted directly into ketones. There is no need to buy MCT oil because coconut is 70-80 percent and has the same impact.

Every day you can start with one teaspoon in the morning and hit 3 teaspoons within a week.

3. External add-on. load.

A lot of studies support the rise in ketosis with regular exercise. It was also found that if you do before meals, the ketone level rises dramatically.

One explanation, in the first few weeks of a low-carb diet starting, it is undesirable to do it.

Why should you choose a keto diet when you clock 50?

The keto diet is for you if you've been yoyoing for years, eat low-fat foods called "diet" or "reduced" without producing results. If you are a person with high cholesterol, high blood pressure, celiac disease, insulin resistance, polycystic ovary syndrome (PCOS) and lack of energy, you may be looking for a keto diet.

Myths of the keto: what the keto is not

Myth # 1: we only eat meat with the keto diet

Most people think the keto diet is the "meat" diet, meaning you're consuming meat morning, noon and evening. Even if you eat more protein and fewer carbs, labeling keto on the "big" diet is probably more accurate. You're going to be eating more fat than you are used to. In fact, about 75 percent of your daily calories in the keto diet would come from healthy fats, 15-20 percent protein. Fat is your combustible!

Foods like butter, bacon, high fat cream, coconut and other oils, salad dressings, cheese, and high-fat yogurt will be your sources of fat. The protein you consume is secondary, but it's important to help you remain in ketosis and burn fat.

Myth # 2: we don't eat vegetables with the keto diet

While up to 80 percent of your calorie intake from healthy fats and 15 percent protein is included in your new way of eating, it does mean the remaining calories will come from carbohydrates. But what carbohydrate type? You have guessed this: vegetables. You'll eat lots of leafy vegetables while avoiding starchy vegetables such as potatoes, corn and carrots. The spinach, lettuce, Swiss chard, kale and cabbage are green leafy vegetables. Hearty squash options such as asparagus, zucchini, cauliflower, and spaghetti do the trick too. Although some foods (such as the whole yogurt) contain minute amounts of carbohydrates (you should still count them), most carbohydrates come from vegetables.

Rich in antioxidants, fiber, and fried eggs, you can continue your day with a green smoothie. Combine a green salad with leafy greens, avocado, olives, blue cheese and grilled salmon for lunch.

In coconut oil, pour in the zucchini and asparagus and grill a steak for dinner. Your meals will be balanced, nutritious and plentiful, and the vegetable fiber is crucial to overall health.

Myth # 3: We don't eat any dessert with the keto diet

Even if it is true that you will no longer consume food and sweets, that is, there will no longer be any sugar in all its forms (cane sugar, corn syrup, honey, agave syrup, maple syrup, etc.), there are natural sweeteners and fruits that will not affect your blood sugar and ketosis goals.

Natural sweeteners like stevia, erythritol, and monk fruit are fine, as are dried berries, cocoa and carob. In reality, it is a great breakfast to add a handful of berries and cocoa powder to a green smoothie! And if after dinner you want dessert, try the fresh berries with soft, homemade stevia whipped cream.

CHAPTER FOUR

List of Foods on the Keto Diet

Lately, the ketogenic diet has become ever more popular. A few studies have found an effective diet low in carbohydrates and high in fat for weight loss, diabetes, and epilepsy.

The ketogenic diet usually restricts to 20-50 grams of carbohydrates per day. While it may seem complicated, there are many nutritious foods that can easily fit into this diet.

Here is a list of foods allowed on a ketogenic diet.

Seafood

Fish and seafood are very suitable foods. B vitamins, potassium, iodine, and selenium are abundant in salmon and other fish. They have hardly any carbohydrates as well.

Shrimp and most crabs do not contain carbohydrates, but we need to limit some shellfish with some carbohydrates.

While these shellfish may still be included in the ketogenic diet, consideration of these carbohydrates is critical when attempting to stay in a tight circle.

Carbohydrate content per 100 grams component of these foods:

- Mussels: 5 grams
- Octopus: 4 grams

- Oysters: 4 grams
- Squid: 3 grams

Salmon, sardine, mackerel, and other fish are very high in omega-3 fatty acids, which are thought to lower insulin levels and increase insulin sensitivity in overweight people.

Low carb vegetables

Starch-free vegetables are low in calories and carbohydrates, but rich in many nutrients, including some minerals and vitamin C. Vegetables and other plants produce fiber not digested by your body and not consumed like other carbohydrates.

Keep in mind that a starchy vegetable serve can provide you well above the day's usual carbohydrate.

Also good for keto diet are vegetables such as cabbage, cauliflower, Brussels sprouts, broccoli, peppers, parsley, lettuce, and more.

Cheese

Cheese is both nutritious and delicious food. If you do not have a healthy reason to avoid cheese, it is a great addition to keto nutrition. (Unfortunately, I can't afford to eat it for health reasons)

There are hundreds of types of cheese, and most are low in carbohydrates.

Avocado

Avocados are extremely useful and appropriate food.

100 grams or about half of an average avocado contains 9 grams of carbohydrates, 7 of which are fiber, so they don't count.

Avocados are high in several vitamins and minerals, including potassium. In addition, avocados can help improve cholesterol and triglyceride levels.

Meat

Meat is considered a staple food in the ketogenic diet.

Fresh meat does not contain carbohydrates (unless injected with various solutions) and is rich in B vitamins and many minerals, including potassium, selenium, and zinc. It is best to consume quality meat from grass-fed animals, but where can one find such a difficult question.

Eggs

Eggs are one of the healthiest and most beneficial foods on the planet. One large egg contains less than 1 gram of carbohydrates and less than 6 grams of protein, which makes eggs an ideal food for a ketogenic lifestyle.

Although egg yolks are high in cholesterol, consuming them does not increase blood cholesterol levels in most people. In fact, eggs show a change in the form of LDL-cholesterol in a way that reduces the risk of cardiovascular disease.

Coconut oil

Coconut oil has unique properties that make it very suitable for a ketogenic diet. To begin with, it contains medium-chain triglycerides (MCT). Unlike long-chain fats, MCTs are used directly in the liver and converted to ketones or used as a fast source of energy. In fact, coconut oil is used to increase ketone levels in people with Alzheimer's disease and other diseases of the brain and nervous system.

Olive oil

Olive oil provides impressive benefits for the heart.

It contains a large amount of oleic acid, a monounsaturated fat that has been found to reduce the risk of heart disease. In addition, cold-pressed olive oil is high in antioxidants.

As a pure source of fat, olive oil does not contain carbohydrates. It is an ideal base for salad sauces and useful mayonnaise.

However, it is not so stable at high temperatures, and it is not good to cook with it.

Nuts

Nuts are a useful high fat and low carb food.

Here are the amounts of digestible carbohydrates in a single dose of 28 grams of nuts:

- Almonds: 3 grams
- Brazil nuts: 1 gram
- Cashew: 8 grams
- Macadamia nuts: 2 grams
- Pecan: 1 gram
- Pistachios: 5 grams
- Nuts: 2 grams
- Chia seeds: 1 gram
- Flax seeds: 0 grams
- Pumpkin seeds: 4 grams
- Sesame: 3 grams

Forest fruits

Now I will not comment on how useful berries are, and I will just say that they are some of the few fruits suitable for the keto diet. They also have lots of fiber, vitamins, and antioxidants.

Butter and cream

If you can tolerate dairy, butter, and cream will be one of your staple foods in your keto diet. They are almost carbohydrate-free and very useful with many fat-soluble vitamins.

Olives

Keep in mind that some olives have more carbohydrates; it is important to follow the labels.

Unsweetened coffee and tea

You can use a carbohydrate-free sweetener such as stevia for sweetening.

Black, keto chocolate

Black chocolate and cocoa are delicious sources of antioxidants.

In fact, cocoa is called "superfruit" because of its rich antioxidant content.

Unsurprisingly, chocolate can be part of a ketogenic diet.

Foods and Diets to Avoid

Which foods to avoid?

A low-carbohydrate diet also called a keto, is one that greatly reduces the intake of carbohydrates. Rather it prefers foods that are high in protein and fat. The general idea is to consume under 50 grams of carbohydrates per day. In this way, the body starts burning for energy proteins and fats which can contribute to weight loss. It is a diet that's perfect for the short term (a couple of months), rather than a few years to pursue.

Carbohydrates are truly in our diet everywhere. At first, remembering all the foods, they're found in can be difficult. On the other side, we are there for you to help! Here are the foods are known to contain a lot of carbohydrates in your diet and how to replace them.

Starchy

The three "P's" (bread, pasta, potatoes) and rice... What's in common with them? We are all very starchy carbohydrates. A healthy alternative to traditional pasta is making pasta from different vegetables, which is pretty easy. Don't hesitate if you are desperate for the bread! Without much effort, you can make keto-bread.

Milk and dairy products

Also, dairy products contain a lot of carbohydrates. That is the case for milk from cow and soy milk. Choose not sweetened almond milk or even coconut milk instead.

Sugar in all its forms

That may be evident, but here we are not only thinking about refined sugar. You should also avoid sugar, maple syrup, and agave nectar. When they have one, all these sugars have little nutritional value. If you have to sweeten your food or drink absolutely consider sucralose or stevia.

The cereals

When we talk about cereals, we don't just mean sweet cereals. Healthy whole wheat cereals also have a high carbohydrate content. To adopt the low-carbohydrate diet guidelines, one should, if at all, eat it in small portions.

Certain fruits and vegetables

Carbohydrates quickly add up in fruits, even if good for your heart. Bananas, raisins, mangoes, pears, dates ... The fruits are all carbohydrates. Citrus fruits, on the other hand, and small berries are no concern.

Beer

Finally, beer is rich in carbohydrates, regardless of the type. Wine, on the other hand, has almost none, and strong alcohol, zero.

Keto Diet Mistakes to Avoid

1. **You eat too much protein and not enough fat.**

A well crafted ketogenic diet does not have a high protein content- it is high in fat. But, eating too much protein can very quickly stop the production of ketone, get you out of nutritional ketosis and lead to what some call "low-carb flu," with symptoms such as general fatigue or loss of energy. Fluctuating, poor mental acuity, etc., and lack of endurance and energy.

The most suitable protein intake for nutritional ketosis seems to be between 1.5 and 1.75 grams per kilogram of ideal body weight per day, higher than the average nutritional intake but not as high as that followed by most fitness enthusiasts who do not adopt a ketogenic diet.

Eating protein stimulates the insulin response and provides amino acids that the body can convert to glucose in the liver. These two things can either decrease, disrupt, or stop the production of the ketone. The anti-ketogenic impact of too much protein intake can worsen if your fat intake is not high enough either; instead of burning fat and ketones, you'll burn the carbohydrates your body makes from protein.

Well-formulated ketogenic diets require at least 80% of the calories provided by dietary fat, most of which must come from high quality saturated and monounsaturated fat. Good quality saturated fats include coconut oil, grass-fed butter, fatty dairy products, or lard, while monounsaturated fats can include olives and olive oil, avocados and l avocado oil, macadamia nuts and animal fats from pasture and pasture. animals raised.

2. You are not eating enough products.

As the ketogenic diet has become more popular outside of its established therapeutic uses, many people can see it as a free pass to start adding butter or MCT oil to their coffee, eating as much bacon. than they want or ban all sources of carbohydrates - including non-starchy vegetables and small amounts of fruit.

This is problematic for several reasons. First, when you limit carbohydrates, your fiber intake generally drops. But fiber is important for preventing constipation, as well as for maintaining a good bacterial balance in your digestive tract.

Second: without an adequate intake of products, it becomes very difficult to consume adequate vitamins, minerals, and antioxidants, essential for cellular functioning and protection against oxidative stress (a byproduct of normal metabolism, especially if you do some exercise).

Whether you are on a ketogenic diet or not, it is best to try to consume large amounts of colorful products, especially leafy vegetables, and other non-starchy vegetables, as well as very colorful fruits like berries. This helps to ensure that you are consuming a lot of fiber and other nutrients essential to your overall health.

If you are following the ketogenic protocol, you will need to tinker with the amounts and sources of products that enter your personal carbohydrate "budget" in order to maintain a normal gut pattern and be well-nourished, while keeping your ketone levels within limits normal. the desired range.

3. You eat less sodium.

Suppose that you have completely switched to consuming the desired amounts and types of carbohydrates, proteins, and fats and that you have successfully limited your carbohydrates to a level that should make you feel energized, focused, and full while you are eating. become "skinny" day by day. Except you don't feel great. Instead, you feel slow, cranky, and your workouts stink. Which give?

When the fast and efficient source of energy you once depended on (carbohydrates) is limited, energy levels can be much lower, at least until your body accelerates fat metabolism. And there are impacts of this change.

As you deplete your internal carbohydrate stores, a significant change in your cellular hydration may occur. For every gram of carbohydrates, you store in your muscles and liver with a normal diet, and you also store three to four grams of water. When you deplete these carbohydrates through low-carbohydrate diets, such as the keto, you lose this water as well as a considerable amount of sodium in the urine, sweat, and breath, because insulin is needed to stimulate kidneys to retain sodium and fluids.

CHAPTER FIVE

How Does Aging Affect Your Nutritional Needs

Eating healthy is a matter of great significance that we are taught as we are young, but there is no other choice when it comes to feeding for the elderly. Nutrition in the elderly requires special features and must follow a pattern that helps improve people's quality of life during this stage of their lives.

For everyone, the value of food is almost the same, but particularly children and the elderly are the ones who should take more care of what they eat since the diet is essential to their health and development. That does not mean, though, that we are neglecting our diet at other stages of life, as what we eat today will take its toll upon us tomorrow.

What should you eat in old age?

It is a question that we all have to ask not only because we live with grandparents or other older relatives at home, but because we're all going to be elderly, and we have to be conscious that an adequate supply for the elderly, working with good health is important.

In order to be healthy, a good diet is necessary, especially when we speak about the elderly. And is that consuming a proper diet will minimize the risk of suffering from some diseases, including arterial, heart, hypertension. Including minerals, proteins, vitamins, fats, carbohydrates, and particularly plenty of water every day is very necessary.

Nutrition for the elderly

Nutritional needs change with the passage of years. Once you begin to leave adulthood, you need a balanced diet in the elderly, in which empty calories should be minimized, and protein, carbohydrates, and vitamins consumed, in addition to ensuring that the food provides good health with calcium, iron and other essential minerals.

Several changes are associated with the passage of age, such as physiological and social effects, which significantly affect the nutritional status of the elderly, and hence their dietary patterns.

Of instance, as teeth are lost, salivation is diminished, and it becomes more difficult to chew food well; also, the senses are no longer the same, they are impaired and thus, there is a chance that interest in food is lost.

To this is added the gradual loss of muscle mass which is associated with a lower demand for energy. Furthermore, we cannot forget that during this stage, it is usual to take medicines that might hinder the absorption of nutrients, so the risk of an older adult is not well-fed triples if all these conditions are not taken into consideration and changes that are experienced during the age.

In the diet from the '50s, the eating habits that had to adapt them to the current biological needs and changes in life need to be checked and updated. For a healthy life after 50 years, it is recommended the highest consumption of fish, poultry, eggs, skimmed meat, legumes, whole grains and nuts, emphasizing that at least half of the proteins consumed are animals and vegetables

Every person interested in or committed to the care of the elderly should be aware of the different diets for the elderly, taking into account some basic aspects and thus finding the most efficient diet. Fats and proteins definitely should be included, but they should be included in their proper measure.

Fats should therefore not exceed 25 percent of the diet, paying particular attention to cooking and limiting the intake of fat items. As for proteins, they must be included in 20%, betting on skimmed dairy products and rising fish intake with the resulting meat reduction.

Fruit, cereals and pasta in 55%, the consumption of certain foods rich in minerals and vitamins are very convenient.

Vegetables and fruits in the diet for the elderly

The elderly diet should include a minimum of two servings of vegetables per day and at least three servings of fruit between meals. Older people's vegetables are important, as they provide the necessary nutrients to help you have a better digestion process and remain healthy.

The vegetables should be cooked and prepared in puree form to promote the chewing process, while the fruits can be eaten naturally if they are very ripe and soft, otherwise in compotes, juices, or smoothies, but without these having processed sugars in the preparation.

Greater consumption of fiber and water

The intestinal passage and the digestion cycle are becoming slower over the years, so constipation symptoms can get more severe. It is therefore advisable to take 25 to 30 grams of fiber per day in conjunction with insoluble and soluble fibers. The insoluble will come from whole grains; whole fruits and vegetables are soluble in fiber.

Additionally, water consumption is essential in any diet, and particularly in the elderly diet. The amount of water in the body decreases during old age, so drinking a minimum of two liters per day, including tea, juices, and broths, is recommended.

Healthy eating for the elderly: 5 or more meals a day

We know that an elderly person's feeding cycle can be complicated many times. The appetite is definitely rising considerably, and one typically eats a third or less of half of what one ate when one is young.

The significance of food variety, preparation process, and amount, which can be eaten every day, is the importance. Organizational shifts in older people's diets are very significant

The food can be divided between 5 or more intakes per day, mixing proteins, fibers, vegetables, cereals, and fruits. Choosing smaller portions more times a day will always be better than the three conventional meals in large portions.

Diet from 50 years and above

It should be avoided that the problem of malnutrition is present during old age, so it is essential that all your nutritional needs are covered. For example:

- Vitamin D: It is vital in nutrition for older people, because a deficit in the consumption of it, can even cause anemia. Slight exposure to the sun, the consumption of fortified cereals, as well as fatty fish, such as salmon, tuna, and mackerel, are ways to absorb this vitamin.
- Vitamin B12: Ideal to continue contributing to the cognitive development of the elderly. They can be consumed in lean meats, fish, and seafood.
- Calcium and phosphorus: They are essential minerals for bones, so their habitual consumption helps to avoid osteoporosis problems . They are consumed in dairy products derived from soybeans, fish and nuts.
- Zinc: It is a natural antioxidant that helps regulate the immune system, so it is important to take it into account. We consume it in meat, fish, eggs, cereals, and legumes.
- Potassium: Helps reduce the risk of hypertension. It is important to reduce sodium intake and increase potassium , which is present in vegetables, yogurts and fruits.
- Fats: The fats that are consumed in a diet for the elderly must constitute 30% of the total calories that an older adult ingests, taking into account that monounsaturated fatty acids should predominate.
- Carbohydrates : In the diets for the elderly, they must contribute 60% of the calories consumed per day. They

must be composed of complex carbohydrates such as rice, pasta, potatoes, cereals, and bread in their integral and fortified versions. As for simple carbohydrates such as sugar, they should try to reduce to the maximum, thus avoiding the consumption of sweets.

Feeding tips in the elderly according to experts

- Feed sometimes, but to get better digestion in smaller quantities.
- Note that cooking a healthy meal is not only necessary but also tasty. With the loss of taste and smell in old age, the taste of food also becomes easy for grandparents to lose. The trick is to reinvent yourself with the food you eat and the way you make them.
- It's also necessary to choose fats correctly. The elderly should avoid greasy desserts and fried foods in the diet.
- Staying active every day is a part of building an old age healthy lifestyle. And muscle strength, bones, and heart can also be improved and will be the perfect complement to a healthy diet in the elderly.

CHAPTER SIX

30-Day Keto Meal Plan for People Over 50

Day 1- Monday

- Breakfast: two-egg fried eggs in butter with slightly spiced spinach.
- Lunch: a burger without rolls with cheese, fried mushrooms, avocados, and a pillow of greens (arugula, baby spinach or mix).
- Dinner: pork chops with braised green beans in coconut oil.

Day 2- Tuesday

- Breakfast: omelet with mushrooms.
- Lunch: salad with tuna, celery, tomatoes and lots of herbs (the same mix salad).
- Dinner: fried or baked chicken in a creamy sauce with stewed broccoli.

Day 3- Wednesday

- Breakfast: bell peppers stuffed with cheese and eggs.
- Lunch: arugula salad with hard-boiled eggs, turkey, avocado, and blue cheese.
- Dinner: grilled salmon with spinach stewed in coconut oil.

Day 4- Thursday

- Breakfast: keto-porridge (chia seeds, flax seeds, hemp seeds, or toasted coconut flakes are used instead of oatmeal) with nuts, a small number of berries and fat cream.
- Lunch: steak with rice and cauliflower, cheese, herbs, avocado, and salsa.
- Dinner: steak with broccoli in cheese sauce.

Day 5- Friday

- Breakfast: boats made from avocado and eggs, baked in the oven.
- Lunch: Caesar salad with chicken.
- Dinner: Pork chops with vegetables.

Day 6- Saturday

- Breakfast: cauliflower toast with cheese and avocado.
- Lunch: Salmon burger with pesto without rolls.
- Dinner: meatballs with zucchini noodles (zoodles) and parmesan.

Day 7-Sunday

- Breakfast: chia seed pudding in coconut milk with nuts.
- Lunch: a salad of greens, eggs, avocados, cheese, and turkey.
- Dinner: coconut curry with chicken (preferably Thai yellow curry paste).

Day 8- Monday

- Breakfast: scrambled eggs, bacon, and tomatoes.
- Lunch: chicken salad with olive oil and feta cheese.
- Dinner: Salmon with asparagus cooked in butter.

Day9- Tuesday

- Breakfast: scrambled eggs with eggs, tomatoes, basil, and goat cheese.
- Lunch: milkshake made from almond milk, peanut butter, cocoa powder, and stevia.
- Dinner: meatballs with vegetables and cheddar cheese.

Day 10- Wednesday

- Breakfast: ketogenic milkshake (½ cup coconut milk, 1 cup any other milk, 2 tablespoons peanut butter, ice and stevia to taste, you can add strawberries).
- Lunch: shrimp salad with olive oil and avocado.
- Dinner: pork chops with parmesan, broccoli, and lettuce.

Day 11- Thursday

- Breakfast: scrambled eggs with avocado, salsa, sweet pepper, onion, and spices of your choice.
- Lunch: celery with guacamole and salsa plus a handful of nuts for dessert.
- Dinner: chicken stuffed with pesto and cream cheese, plus vegetables.

Day 12- Friday

- Breakfast: sugar-free yogurt with peanut butter, cocoa powder, and stevia.
- Lunch: beef fried in coconut oil with vegetables.
- Dinner: a burger without rolls with bacon, egg, and cheese.

Day 13- Saturday

- Breakfast: omelet with ham, cheese, and vegetables.
- Lunch: sliced ham and cheese in a bite with nuts.
- Dinner: white fish (for Ambala, halibut, tilapia, cod, white salmon, hake), spinach, eggs, and cooked in coconut oil.

Day14- Sunday

- Breakfast: fried eggs with bacon and mushrooms.
- Lunch: a burger without rolls with salsa, cheese, and guacamole.
- Dinner: steak, eggs, and salad.

Day 15 – Monday

- Breakfast: two boiled eggs.

- Lunch: salad with walnuts, cheese, and beef, chicken broth.
- Dinner: cabbage rolls with beef.

Day 16- Tuesday

- Breakfast: scrambled eggs with ham
- Lunch: mushrooms with cheese, green salad
- Dinner: cottage cheese pancakes with sour cream

Day 17- Wednesday

- Breakfast: toast with peanut butter.
- Lunch: fish ear.
- Dinner: meat salad.

Day 18- Thursday

- Breakfast: cottage cheese
- Lunch: chicken broth, boiled egg
- Dinner: beef entrecote, green vegetable salad with butter

Day 19 – Friday

- Breakfast: fried eggs from 2 eggs.
- Lunch: baked chicken, greens.
- Dinner: cheese, pancakes from zucchini.

Day 20- Saturday

- Breakfast: ham and cheese toast
- Lunch: fish cutlet, tomato, and cucumber salad
- Dinner: Pork chop, greens

Day 21- Sunday

- Breakfast: omelet of 3 eggs
- Lunch: meat lunch, brown rice
- Dinner: redfish baked, vegetables

Day 22- Monday

- Breakfast: two-egg fried eggs in butter with slightly spiced spinach.
- Lunch: a burger without rolls with cheese, fried mushrooms, avocados, and a pillow of greens (arugula, baby spinach or mix).
- Dinner: pork chops with braised green beans in coconut oil.

Day 23- Tuesday

- Breakfast: omelet with mushrooms.
- Lunch: salad with tuna, celery, tomatoes and lots of herbs (the same mix salad).
- Dinner: fried or baked chicken in a creamy sauce with stewed broccoli.

Day 24- Wednesday

- Breakfast: bell peppers stuffed with cheese and eggs.
- Lunch: arugula salad with hard-boiled eggs, turkey, avocado, and blue cheese.
- Dinner: grilled salmon with spinach stewed in coconut oil.

Day 25- Thursday

- Breakfast: cottage cheese
- Lunch: chicken broth, boiled egg
- Dinner: beef entrecote, green vegetable salad with butter

Day 26 – Friday

- Breakfast: fried eggs from 2 eggs.

- Lunch: baked chicken, greens.
- Dinner: cheese, pancakes from zucchini.

Day 27- Saturday

- Breakfast: ham and cheese toast
- Lunch: fish cutlet, tomato, and cucumber salad
- Dinner: Pork chop, greens

Day 28- Sunday

- Breakfast: omelet of 3 eggs
- Lunch: meat lunch, brown rice
- Dinner: redfish baked, vegetables

Day 29- Monday

- Breakfast: two-egg fried eggs in butter with slightly spiced spinach.
- Lunch: a burger without rolls with cheese, fried mushrooms, avocados, and a pillow of greens (arugula, baby spinach or mix).
- Dinner: pork chops with braised green beans in coconut oil.

Day 30- Tuesday

- Breakfast: omelet with mushrooms.
- Lunch: salad with tuna, celery, tomatoes and lots of herbs (the same mix salad).
- Dinner: fried or baked chicken in a creamy sauce with stewed broccoli.

CHAPTER SEVEN

Simple Keto Recipes

- **Breakfast**

1. The classic keto-style bacon with eggs

Ingredients

- 8 eggs
- 150 g bacon, sliced
- cherry tomato (optional)
- fresh parsley (optional)

Instructions

- Fry the bacon until it is crispy. Set aside on a plate.
- Fry the eggs in the bacon fat the way you like it. Cut the cherry tomatoes in half and fry them at the same time.
- Salpimentar to taste.

2. Crispy Cheese Keto Omelette

Ingredients

Omelet

- 2 eggs
- 2 tbsp whipping cream
- salt and ground black pepper
- 1 tbsp butter or coconut oil
- 75 g grated or sliced cheese, cured

Filling

- 2 sliced mushrooms
- 2 sliced cherry tomatoes
- 2 tbsp (30 g) cream cheese
- 15 g spinach sprouts
- 30 g turkey cold cuts
- 1 tsp dried oregano

Instructions

- In a bowl, beat the eggs, cream, salt, and pepper.
- Heat a tablespoon of butter in a nonstick skillet over medium heat. Spread the cheese evenly in the pan so that it covers the entire bottom. Fry over medium heat until bubbly.

- Carefully incorporate the egg mixture over the cheese and reduce heat – Cook a few minutes without stirring.
- Fill half with mushrooms, tomatoes, spinach, cream cheese, turkey, and oregano – Fry a few more minutes.
- When the egg mixture begins to set (it can still be quite loose on top, but not too much), turn the empty half over half with the ingredients, forming a half-moon. Fry a few more minutes and enjoy!

3. Ketogenic stuffed mushrooms

Ingredients

- 12 mushrooms
- 225 g bacon
- 2 tbsp Butter
- 200 g (200 ml) cream cheese
- 3 tbsp fresh chives, finely chopped
- 1 tsp Spanish paprika
- salt and pepper

Preparation

- Preheat the oven to 200 ° C.
- Stir in the bacon until crisp. Allow to cool and process to crumble. Save fat from the bacon

- Remove the stalk from the mushroom and chop finely. Stir in the fat and add butter if necessary.
- Put mushrooms in an oiled frying pan.
- In a bowl, crushed bacon with fried mushroom stalk and mix the remaining ingredients. Fill each mushroom with a small amount of mixture.
- Bake for 20 minutes or until the mushrooms are brown.

4. Keto cured salmon with scrambled eggs and chives

Ingredients

- 2 eggs
- 2 tbsp Butter
- 60 ml whipping cream
- 1 tbsp fresh chives, chopped
- 50 g cured salmon
- salt and pepper

Instructions

- Beat the eggs well. Melt the butter in a pan. Add the cream and heat carefully while stirring.
- Simmer the mixture for a few minutes while constantly stirring so that the eggs are creamy.

- Season with chopped chives, salt, and freshly ground pepper. Serve with several slices of cured salmon .

5. Keto fried eggs with kale and pork

Ingredients

- 225 g kale
- 75 g butter
- 175 g smoked pork bacon or bacon
- 60 ml frozen blueberries
- 30 g (75 ml) pecans or nuts
- 4 eggs
- salt and pepper

Instructions

- Cut and chop the kale into large squares (pre-washed kale is an excellent shortcut). Melt two-thirds of the butter in a pan and fry the kale quickly over high heat until it browns a little around the edges.
- Remove the kale from the pan and set aside. Brown the bacon or pork bacon in the same pan until they are crispy.
- Lower the heat. Put the sauteed kale back in the pan and add the blueberries and nuts. Stir until hot — Reserve in a bowl.

- Raise the heat and fry the eggs in the rest of the butter. Salpimentar to taste place two fried eggs with each serving of vegetables and serve immediately.

6. Omelet Caprese

Ingredients

- 2 tbsp olive oil
- 6 eggs
- 100 g cherry tomatoes, cut in halves or tomatoes cut into slices
- 1 tbsp fresh basil or dried basil
- 150 g (325 ml) fresh mozzarella cheese
- salt and pepper

Instructions

1. Break the eggs in a bowl to mix and add salt and black pepper to taste. Beat well with a fork until everything is completely mixed. Add basil and stir.
2. Cut the tomatoes into halves or slices. Chop or slice the cheese.

3. Heat the oil in a large skillet. Fry the tomatoes for a few minutes.
4. Pour the egg mixture over the tomatoes. Wait until it becomes a little firm and add the cheese.
5. Lower the heat and let the omelet harden. Serve immediately, and enjoy!

7. Scrambled eggs

Ingredients

- 2 eggs
- 30 g butter
- Salt and ground black pepper

Instructions

1. Beat the eggs together with some salt and pepper using a fork.
2. Melt the butter in a nonstick skillet over medium heat. Look closely: butter does not turn golden!
3. Pour the eggs into the pan and mix for 1-2 minutes until they are creamy and cooked a little less than you like. Remember that the eggs will continue to cook even once you put them on your plate.

Tips!

- These creamy eggs, pair well with many popular low carb dishes. Of course, there is the option of eating them with classic accompaniments such as bacon or sausage, but there are other great options such as salmon, avocado, cold cuts and cheese (cheddar, fresh mozzarella or feta).
- And if you're very hungry (or are cooking with large eggs), do not be shy: use more butter!

8. Chocolate Chia Pudding With Warm Pear

Ingredients

- 200 ml Plant drink (soy)
- 20 g Nutri-Plus Shape & Shake Chocolate
- 15 g Chia seeds
- 1 pear
- 5 g coconut oil
- something Vanilla and cinnamon

Preparation

Preparation time: 10 minutes plus cooling time

At best, prepare this recipe the night before, so that the Chiapudding can swell in peace.

1. Put the plant drink in a blender jar and add the Shape & Shake protein powder.
2. Mix both together vigorously until no lumps are left.
3. Now add the Chia seeds and stir them, so they can swell in peace. Stir in the first hour between times, so that everything spreads well and the shake can be taken anywhere from the Chia seeds.
4. Leave the chia pudding in the fridge overnight.
5. Cut the pear down and heat some coconut oil in a small pot.
6. Add the pieces of pear to the pot and let it simmer for 2-3 minutes. Vanilla and cinnamon to it and already the pears to Chia pudding.

9. Scrambled eggs in a cup

Ingredients

- 2 eggs
- 2 tbsp cream to beat
- salt and pepper
- 1 tbsp Butter

Instructions

1. Grease a large cup or bowl with mild butter. Beat the eggs and the cream to beat. Fill the cup to a maximum of two thirds, as the eggs will gain volume when cooked.
2. Add a pinch of salt and freshly ground black pepper or cayenne.
3. Cook in the microwave at maximum power for 1-2 minutes (700 watts). Stir and microwave another minute. Keep in mind that the eggs are still made after removing them from the heat, so do not overdo them.
4. Remove and add a little butter. Allow cooling for one minute.

10. Ketogenic frittata of goat cheese and mushrooms

Ingredients

- Frittata
- 150 g mushrooms
- 75 g fresh spinach
- 50 g chives
- 50 g butter
- 6 eggs
- 110 g goat cheese
- Salt and ground black pepper
- At your service
- 150 g green leafy vegetables
- 2 tbsp olive oil
- Salt and ground black pepper

Instructions

1. Preheat the oven to 175 ° C (350 ° F).
2. Grate or crumble the cheese and mix in a bowl with the eggs. Salt and pepper to taste.
3. Cut the mushrooms into small pieces. Chop the chives.
4. Melt the butter over medium heat in a pan suitable for the oven and fry the mushrooms and onions for 5-10 minutes or until golden brown.
5. Add the spinach to the pan and fry for another 1-2 minutes. Pepper.

6. Pour the egg mixture in the pan. Bake for about 20 minutes or until browned and firm in the middle.
7. Serve with green leafy vegetables and olive oil.

11. Vegan Scrambled Eggs With Silk Tofu

Ingredients

- 300 g silken tofu
- 100 g Tofu, tight
- 30 g Nutri-Plus Protein Powder Neutral
- 1 small one onion
- A good pinch Kala namak
- Something Salt, pepper, turmeric
- Fresh chives
- 1-2 tbsp neutral vegetable oil

Preparation

Preparation time: 20 minutes

1. Put the silk tofu, the protein powder, turmeric, Kala Namak, salt and pepper together in a blender jar and mix well with the blender.
2. Now crumb the firm tofu, cut the onion into small cubes and put them under the silk tofu mixture.
3. Heat some oil in a pan and add the mass for the vegan scrambled egg.
4. Slowly set it to a medium level and stir again and again.
5. Give the scrambled eggs, some time, it takes a little longer than the original! But the wait is worth it.
6. Once the desired consistency is achieved, you can fold in some fresh chives and enjoy your vegan scrambled eggs.

12 bLow carb beef roll

Recipe

- 900 g ground beef
- 1/2 tsp fine Himalayan salt
- tsp black pepper
- 1/4 cup yeast
- large eggs
- tbsp avocado oil
- 1 tbsp lemon zest

- 1/4 cup chopped parsley
- 1/4 cup chopped fresh oregano
- cloves of garlic

Cooking

- Preheat the oven to 204 degrees.
- In a large bowl, combine ground beef, salt, black pepper, and nutritional yeast.
- In a blender or food processor, beat eggs, butter, herbs, and garlic. Beat until eggs begin to froth, and then add chopped herbs, lemon zest, and garlic.
- Add the egg mixture to the minced meat and mix.
- Pour the meat mixture into a small 8 x 4-inch dish. Smooth well.
- Put on the middle rack and bake for 50-60 minutes, until the top turns golden brown.
- Carefully remove from the oven and tilt the mold over the sink to drain all the liquid. Allow cooling for 5-10 minutes before slicing.
- Garnish with fresh lemon and serve.

14 Crispy Ginger Mackerel with Vegetables

Recipe

Marinade:

- tbsp grated ginger
- 1 tbsp lemon juice
- tbsp olive oil
- 1 tbsp coconut amino acids
- Salt and pepper to taste

Fish:

- 2 (about 226 g) boneless mackerel filet
- 28 g almonds
- ½ cup broccoli
- tbsp oils
- ½ small yellow onion
- 1/3 cup diced red bell pepper
- small sun-dried tomatoes (chopped)
- tbsp mashed avocado

Cooking

- Preheat the oven to 204 ° C. Place a baking sheet on parchment paper or foil.
- Combine grated ginger, lemon juice, olive oil, coconut amino acids, and a little salt and pepper. Grate the mackerel fillet with half the marinade.

- Place the fillet on a baking sheet with the skin up. Bake for 12-15 minutes or until the skin becomes crisp.
- Place the almonds on a separate baking sheet. Cook for 5-6 minutes or until the nuts turn brown. Remove from the oven and cool before chopping.
- Lightly steam the broccoli until it begins to soften, but becomes soft. Cut into pieces.
- Heat the pan over medium heat, then add the oil and let it melt. Sauté the onions and peppers until they are soft.
- Add broccoli and sun-dried tomatoes, and continue cooking until they heat up.
- Turn off the heat, then mix with the rest of the dressing and roasted almonds. Serve with the avocado smoothie.

15 Spinach Egg Casserole

Recipe

- 283.5 g spinach
- ¼ chopped onion
- minced garlic
- 56.7 g cream cheese
- 59.5 ml buttercream
- 1 tbsp butter

- 1/8 tsp ground nutmeg
- eggs
- Salt and pepper to taste
- 1 tbsp grated Parmesan cheese

Cooking

- Boil water in a pan, add salt and spinach and simmer for 1 minute. Drain the spinach, squeeze, chop and set aside.
- Heat the oil in a pan, add chopped onion and garlic, and cook for 3 minutes or until it becomes aromatic. Add cream cheese and heavy cream, and cook until smooth.
- Add chopped spinach and cook for 10 minutes. Season with nutmeg, salt, and pepper.
- Preheat the oven to 204 degrees.
- Put the spinach in a baking dish and make small indentations with the back of the spoon.
- Break into each hole in the egg.
- Bake for up to 15 minutes or until egg whites is cooked.
- Season the casserole with salt and pepper. Serve sprinkled with grated Parmesan cheese.

➢ Lunch recipes

16 Fish in tomato sauce

Ingredients

- 4 frozen white fish fillets of your choice
- 2 cups cherry tomatoes cut in half
- 2 finely sliced garlic cloves
- 120 ml light chicken broth
- 60 ml of dry white wine (or use more chicken stock)
- 1/2 teaspoon salt
- 1/2 teaspoon black pepper
- 1/4 cup finely chopped fresh basil leaves (to garnish)

Preparation

- Place the tomatoes, garlic, salt, and pepper in a pan over medium heat. Cook for 5 minutes or until tomatoes are soft.
- Add chicken broth, white wine (if used), frozen fish fillets, and chopped basil. Cover and simmer 20-25 minutes, until the fish is fully cooked.
- Finally, sprinkle with an additional handful of chopped basil and serve on a bed of rice, couscous or quinoa, if desired.

Note: Thick white fish fillets such as cod, halibut, catfish, or mahi-mahi work best for this recipe.

17 Sea Bass and Peppers Salad

Ingredients

- Seabass was very clean: A fillet of 150 g.
- Assorted lettuces: 100 g.
- Chives: To taste
- Fresh or roasted red pepper: 1
- Cherry tomatoes To taste
- Garlic clove and parsley 1
- Leek 1
- Carrot 1
- Olive oil One tablespoon
- Salt and lemon to taste

Directions

1. We put the fillet of sea bass in aluminum foil. In the mortar, chop the garlic and parsley, add 2 small teaspoons of oil and cover the fillet of sea bass with it.
2. We also put some leek and carrot strips on the sea bass fillet (the vegetable ribbons can be made with the fruit peeler) and a little salt. Now we close the foil tightly and

take it into the oven at 120 ºC for 8-10 minutes. Once cooked, let it cool.

3. In a salad bowl, we put the lettuce mixture and chop the chives and pepper very finely. We add it too. Add the cherry tomatoes cut into quarters. Add only a small teaspoon of olive oil, salt, and lemon as a dressing and stir well and now add the fish with the vegetables that we have cooked in the oven and ready to eat

18 Mexican baked beans and rice

Ingredients

- 5 ml (1 teaspoon) unsalted butter
- 1 chopped yellow onion
- 3/4 cup (190 mL) basmati rice
- 5 ml (1 teaspoon) ground cumin
- 1 seeded jalapeño pepper
- 300 ml (1 1/4 cups) chicken stock
- 125 ml (1/2 cup) tomato sauce
- 3/4 cup (190 mL) canned black kidney beans
- 30 ml (2 tablespoons) finely chopped parsley
- 1 lime
- Salt and pepper, to taste

Preparation

1. In a saucepan, melt the butter and add the onion. Simmer.
2. Add the rice and ground cumin. Continue cooking for about 2 minutes. Add the Jalapeno pepper. Deglaze with chicken stock and season.
3. Add the tomato sauce — cover and cook over medium heat for about 12 minutes.
4. When the rice is cooked, add the black beans and parsley. Continue cooking for minutes.
5. Add lime juice, salt, pepper, and serve.

19 Easy Baked Shepherd Pie

Ingredients

- 500 grams of freshly ground duck meat
- 3 tablespoons oil or olive oil
- 1 small onion, finely chopped
- 1 tsp ready-made garlic and salt seasoning
- 1 tablespoon dry spice chimichurri
- 4 medium cooked and mashed potatoes
- 1 tablespoon full of butter
- 100 ml of milk
- 25 grams of grated Parmesan cheese

- 1 pinch of salt

Preparation

1. In a pan heat oil, onion, and fry.
2. Add the meat and garlic and salt seasoning.
3. Fry well until the accumulated meat water dries.
4. After the meat is fried, add enough water to cover the meat.
5. Let it cook with the pan without a lid until the water almost dries again.
6. Add the chimichurri, stir and cook until the water dries, and the meat is fried until well dried.
7. Put the meat in an ovenproof dish and set aside.
8. Prepare a mash by mixing the remaining ingredients and spread over the meat.
9. Bake for about 20 minutes or until flushed.
10. Remove and serve.

20 Fish in the herb, garlic, and tomato sauce

Ingredients

- 6 teeth garlic peeled and whole

- 300 grams of halved mini onion
- 300 grams of halved pear (or cherry) tomato
- 1 packet of herbs (basil, parsley, and thyme) coarsely chopped
- 1/2 cup of olive oil
- 1 merluza fillet
- 2 cups wheat flour
- 3 egg
- 3 cups cornmeal
- black pepper to taste
- frying oil
- salt to taste

Preparation

1. In a large baking dish, place the garlic, onion, tomato, and herbs. Mix the olive oil, salt, and pepper.
2. Wrap the fish fillets and cover them with plastic wrap.
3. Refrigerate and marinate for 1 hour.
4. Remove the fish fillets, pass in the flour, then in the eggs beaten with a little salt and last in the cornmeal. Refrigerate.
5. Put the baking sheet with the marinade in the oven, preheated to 200 ° C, and let it bake for about 20 minutes.
6. Remove the breaded fillets from the refrigerator and fry them in hot oil until golden brown.

7. Serve the fish with the sauce in the baking dish.

21 Hot Salad with Kale and White Beans

Ingredients:

- 1 large bunch of kale well washed
- 1-2 tablespoons olive oil
- 1 stem of fresh rosemary, with the leaves removed from the stem and cut
- 1 small onion, cut
- 1 large carrot, sliced
- ½ teaspoon finely grated lemon zest
- 1 clove garlic, minced
- Salt to taste
- 2 cups cooked lima beans or other white beans plus cooking broth or 1 can (14 ounces)
- 1 cup plain parsley, cut
- Extra virgin olive oil, to spray
- Juice from ½ to small lemon, to spray (optional)

Preparation

1. Remove the leaves from the kale stalks. Cut into bite-sized pieces. Set aside.

2. Drain the white beans, reserving their broth. If you use canned beans, drain and wash. Set aside.
3. In a large pot, heat the oil over medium-high heat until it starts to boil. Add the rosemary, reserving a teaspoon, let it boil for a moment, and then add the chopped onion, carrot, and lemon zest. Mix well and reduce the temperature. Cover and "sweat" the vegetables for minutes or until they are soft and the onion is a little golden, occasionally stirring to make sure they do not stick or burn.
4. Increase the temperature to medium-high. Add the cut garlic, stir and cook for 5 minutes. Add the cut greens with a good pinch of salt and sauté until they begin to wilt and soften.
5. Add ½ cup of the bean or water broth. Bring to a boil, lower the temperature for 10 to 15 minutes, or until the greens are soft and the liquid has evaporated. Put a little more broth or water if the vegetables seem very dry.
6. Mix the chopped parsley and the remaining teaspoon of rosemary, cook for 1 minute, then add the beans to the pot. Mix carefully with the greens. Try the seasoning.
7. Put off the burner and let the quinoa stand covered for 5 minutes. Serve sprinkled with a little olive oil and some lemon juice.

22 Scallion Swordfish

Ingredients

- 800 g of swordfish
- 1 lemon (medium)
- 1 dl of olive oil
- 2 Onions
- 1 dl of White Wine
- 1 c. (dessert) chopped parsley
- 4 royal gala apples
- 1 c. (soup) Butter
- 150 g chives
- Salt q.s.
- Paprika q.s.
- Salsa q.s.

Preparation

1. Season the swordfish slices with salt and lemon juice. Let them marinate for 30 minutes. After this time, fry them in olive oil. Add the peeled and sliced onions to half-moons and let them sauté.
2. Cool with white wine and season with a little more salt. Sprinkle with chopped parsley. Peel the apples cut them into wedges and sauté them in butter. Peel the spring onions and add them to the fruit.

3. Season with some salt and paprika. Serve the fish topped with the spring onions and accompanied with the sauteed apple and spring onions. Garnish with parsley.

23 Sharpened Lamb Shoulder (Keto)

Ingredients

- 3 tbsp olive oil
- 4 minced cloves of garlic
- tbsp dried mint
- tsp ground cinnamon
- tsp ground caraway seeds
- tsp salt
- ½ tsp ground chili
- Lemon zest and 1 lemon juice
- Lamb shoulder (about 1.8 kg)

Cooking

- In a small bowl, put all the ingredients except lamb. Mix well.
- Make deep cuts across the lamb's shoulder and rub it with the cooked marinade.

- Refrigerate for at least 4 hours, preferably at night.
- Preheat the oven to 150 degrees.
- Put the lamb on a large roasting pan and cook for 5-5.5 hours, covering it with aluminum foil after the first hour. Cook until the meat exfoliates from the bone.
- Remove from the oven and let stand for 20 minutes.
- Cut into slices and serve hot along with mashed cauliflower and low-carb sauce.

24 Keto Shepherd's Pie

Ingredients

- 2 tbsp butter
- 450 g minced lamb
- ½ medium yellow onion, chopped
- 3 minced garlic cloves
- ½ cup minced celery
- 2 tbsp sugar-free tomato paste
- 1 tbsp Worcestershire sauce
- ½ cup chicken stock
- ¼ cup dry red wine
- ½ tsp xanthan gum
- 680 g "cauliflower" rice

- 1 cup oily whipped cream
- 1 cup grated cheddar cheese
- ¼ cup grated parmesan
- 1 tsp dried thyme

Cooking

- Preheat the oven to 176 degrees. Heat oil in a large skillet.
- Put minced meat, onion, garlic, celery, tomato paste, Worcestershire sauce, red wine and chicken stock in a pan.
- Cook until the meat is lightly browned and the vegetables soft. Sprinkle with xanthan gum and mix.
- Put cauliflower rice, greasy whipped cream, cheddar cheese, parmesan and thyme in a food processor. Mix until cauliflower turns into a smoothie.
- Put the meat mixture in a baking dish, and on top lay the mashed cauliflower.
- Bake the cake for 45 minutes or until it is browned on top. Let cool for 10 minutes and serve.

25 Low Carb Shakshuka

Recipe

- tbsp avocado oil
- 2 red bell peppers diced

- ½ medium yellow onion, chopped
- 3 cups chopped cabbage
- 2 tsp seasoning harissa
- 2 tsp garlic powder
- 2 tsp caraway seeds
- ½ tsp sea salt
- 2 tbsp low carb tomato paste
- 2 tbsp water
- 4 large eggs

Cooking

- Heat the avocado oil in a large skillet over medium heat.
- Add bell peppers and white onions, and sauté for 5 minutes.
- Add cabbage and spices, then tomato paste and water, stirring until smooth. Cook for another 5 minutes, then reduce heat.
- Make four recesses with a spoon and break into each egg. Sprinkle with salt and cook under the lid for 5 minutes or until the eggs are ready.
- Divide into four servings, put a keto-friendly spicy sauce on top and serve.

- Dinner recipes

17 Cauliflower and Pumpkin Casserole

Ingredients

- 2 tbsp. olive oil
- 1/4 medium yellow onion, minced
- 6 cups chopped forage kale into small pieces (about 140 g)
- 1 little clove garlic, minced
- Salt and freshly ground black pepper
- 1/2 cup low sodium chicken broth
- 2 cups of 1.5 cm diced pumpkin (about 230 g)
- 2 cups of 1.5 cm diced zucchini (about 230 g)
- 2 tbsp. mayonnaise
- 3 cups frozen, thawed brown rice
- 1 cup grated Swiss cheese
- 1/3 cup grated Parmesan
- 1 cup panko flour
- 1 large beaten egg
- Cooking spray

Preparation

1. Preheat oven to 200 ° C. Heats the oil in a large nonstick skillet over medium heat. Add onions and cook, occasionally stirring, until browned and tender (about 5 minutes). Add the cabbage, garlic, and 1/2 teaspoon salt and 1/2 teaspoon pepper and cook until the cabbage is light (about 2 minutes).
2. Add the stock and continue to cook until the cabbage withers, and most of the stock evaporates (about 5 minutes). Add squash, zucchini, and 1/2 teaspoon salt and mix well. Continue cooking until the pumpkin begins to soften (about 8 minutes). Remove from heat and add mayonnaise.
3. In a bowl, combine cooked vegetables, brown rice, cheese, 1/2 cup flour, and large egg and mix well. Spray a 2-liter casserole with cooking spray. Spread the mixture across the bottom of the pan and cover with the remaining flour, 1/4 teaspoon salt and a few pinches of pepper. Bake until the squash and zucchini are tender and the top golden and crispy (about 35 minutes). Serve hot.

Advance Preparation Tip: Freeze the casserole for up to 2 weeks. Cover with aluminum foil and heat at 180 ° C until warm (35 to 45 minutes).

18 Thai beef salad Tears of the Tiger

Ingredients

- 800 g of beef tenderloin
- For the marinade :
- 2 tablespoons of soy sauce
- 1 tablespoon soup of honey
- 1 pinch of the pepper mill
- For the sauce :
- 1 small bunch of fresh coriander
- 1 small bouquet of mint
- 3 tablespoons soup of fish sauce
- lemon green
- 1 clove of garlic
- tablespoons soup of sugar palm (or brown sugar)
- 1 bird pepper or ten drops of Tabasco
- 1 small glass of raw Thai rice to make grilled rice powder
- 200 g of arugula or young shoots of salad

Preparation

- Cut the beef tenderloin into strips and put it in a container. Sprinkle with 2 tablespoons soy sauce, 1 tablespoon honey, and pepper. Although soak thoroughly and let marinate 1 hour at room temperature.

- Meanwhile, prepare the roasted rice powder. Pour a glass of Thai rice into an anti-adhesive pan. Dry color the rice, constantly stirring to avoid burning. When it has a lovely color, get rid of it on a plate and let it cool.
- When it has cooled, reduce it to powder by mixing it with the robot.
- Wash and finely chop mint and coriander. Put in a container and add lime juice, chopped garlic clove, 3 tablespoons Nuoc mam, 3 tablespoons brown sugar, 3 tablespoons water, 1 tablespoon sauce soy, and a dozen drops of Tabasco. Mix well and let stand the time that the sugar melts and the flavors mix.
- Place a bed of salad on a dish. Cook the beef strips put them on the salad. Sprinkle with the spoonful of sauce and roasted rice powder. To be served as is or with a Thai cooked white rice scented.

19 Stuffed apples with shrimp

Ingredients

- 6 medium apples
- 1 lemon juice
- 2 tablespoons butter

Filling:

- 300 gr of shrimp
- 1 onion minced
- ½ cup chopped parsley
- 2 tbsp flour
- 1 can of cream/cream
- 100 gr of curd
- 1 tablespoon butter
- 1 tbsp pepper sauce
- Salt to taste

Preparation

- Cut a cap from each apple, remove the seeds a little from the pulp on the sides, and put the pulp in the bottom, but leaving a cavity.
- Pass a little lemon and some butter on the apples, bake them in the oven. Remove from oven, let cool and bring to freeze.
- Prepare the shrimp sauce in a pan by mixing the butter with the flour, onion, parsley, and pepper sauce.
- Then add the prawn shrimp to the sauce. When boiling, mix the cream cheese and sour cream.

- Stuff each apple. Serve hot or cold, as you prefer.

20 A Quick Recipe of Grilled Chicken Salad with Oranges

Ingredients:

- 75 ml (1/3 cup) orange juice
- 30 ml (2 tablespoons) lemon juice
- 45 ml (3 tablespoons) of extra virgin olive oil
- 15 ml (1 tablespoon) Dijon mustard
- 2 cloves of garlic, chopped
- 1 ml (1/4 teaspoon) salt, or as you like
- Freshly ground pepper to your taste
- 1 lb. (450 g) skinless chicken breast, trimmed
- 25 g (1/4 cup) pistachio or flaked almonds, toasted
- 600 g (8c / 5 oz) of mesclun, rinsed and dried
- 75 g (1/2 cup) minced red onion
- 2 medium oranges, peeled, quartered and sliced

Preparation:

- Place the orange juice, lemon juice, oil, mustard, garlic, salt, and pepper in a small bowl or jar with an airtight lid; whip or shake to mix. Reserve 75 milliliters (1/3 cup) of this salad vinaigrette and 45 milliliters (three tablespoons) for basting.

- Place the rest of the vinaigrette in a shallow glass dish or resealable plastic bag. Add the chicken and turn it over to coat. Cover or close and marinate in the refrigerator for at least 20 minutes or up to two hours.
- Preheat the barbecue over medium heat. Lightly oil the grill by rubbing it with a crumpled paper towel soaked in oil (use the tongs to hold the paper towel). Remove the chicken from the marinade and discard the marinade. Grill the chicken 10 to 15 centimeters (four to six inches) from the heat source, basting the cooked sides with the basting vinaigrette, until it is no longer pink in the center, and Instant-read thermometer inserted in the thickest part records 75 ° C (170 ° F), four to six minutes on each side. Transfer the chicken to a cutting board and let it rest for five minutes.
- Meanwhile, grill almonds (or pistachios) in a small, dry pan on medium-low heat, stirring constantly, until lightly browned, about two to three minutes. Transfer them to a bowl and let them cool.
- Place the salad and onion mixture in a large bowl. Mix with the vinaigrette reserved for the salad. Divide the salad into four plates. Slice chicken and spread on salads. Sprinkle orange slices on top and sprinkle with pistachios (or almonds).

21 Red Curry with Vegetable

Ingredients

- 600 g sweet potatoes
- 200 g canned chickpeas
- 2 leek whites
- 2 tomatoes
- 100 g of spinach shoots
- 40 cl of coconut milk
- 1 jar of Greek yogurt
- 1 lime
- 3 cm fresh ginger
- 1 small bunch of coriander
- 1/2 red onion
- 2 cloves garlic
- 4 tbsp. red curry paste
- salt

Preparation

- Peel the sweet potatoes and cut them into pieces. Clean the leek whites and cut them into slices. Peel and seed the tomatoes.

- Mix the Greek yogurt with a drizzle of lime juice, chopped onion, salt, and half of the coriander leaves.
- In a frying pan, heat 15 cl of coconut milk until it reduces and forms a multitude of small bubbles. Brown curry paste with chopped ginger and garlic.
- Add vegetables, drained chickpeas, remaining coconut milk, and salt. Cook for 20 min covered, then 5 min without lid for the sauce to thicken.
- When serving, add spinach sprouts and remaining coriander. Serve with the yogurt sauce.

22 Baked Turkey Breast with Cranberry Sauce

Ingredients

- 2 kilos of whole turkey breast
- 1 tablespoon olive oil
- 1/4 cup onion
- 2 cloves of garlic
- thyme
- poultry seasonings
- you saved
- coarse-grained salt
- 2 butter spoons

- 1/4 cup minced echallot
- 1/4 cup chopped onion
- 1 clove garlic
- 2 tablespoons flour
- 1 1/2 cups of blueberries
- 2 cups apple cider
- 2 tablespoons maple honey
- peppers

Preparation

1. Grind in the blender ¼ cup onion, 2 garlic with herbs. Add 1 tablespoon of oil and spread the breast with this.
2. Put in the baking tray, add a cup of citron and bake at 350 Fahrenheit (180 ° C) to have a thermometer record 165 Fahrenheit (75 ° C) inside, about an hour, add ½ cup of water if necessary.
3. Bring the citron to a boil, add the blueberries, and leave a few minutes. In the butter (2 tablespoons), acitronar the onion (1/4 cup), echallot, and garlic (1 clove).
4. Add the flour to the onion and echallot and leave a few minutes. Add the citron, cranberries, and honey and leave on low heat. Season with salt and pepper, let the blueberries are soft, go to the processor, and if you want to strain.
5. Return to the fire and let it thicken slightly.

6. Slice the thin turkey breast and serve with the blueberry sauce.

32 Italian Keto Casserole

Ingredients

- 200 g Shirataki noodles
- 2 tbsp olive oil
- 1 small onion, diced
- 2 garlic cloves, finely chopped
- 1 tsp dried marjoram
- 450 g ground beef
- 1 tsp salt
- ½ tsp ground pepper
- 2 chopped tomatoes
- 1 cup of fat cream
- 340 g ricotta cheese
- ⅓ cup grated parmesan
- 1 egg
- ¼ cup parsley, roughly chopped

Cooking

- Preheat the oven to 190 degrees.

- Prepare the shirataki noodles as indicated on the packaging, strain well and set aside.
- Place a large non-stick pan over high heat. Add oil, onion, garlic, and marjoram, and fry for 2-3 minutes, until the onion is soft.
- Add ground beef, salt and pepper, and simmer, stirring, while the mixture is browned (if it is watery, drain the excess liquid).
- Add tomatoes and fat cream, and cook for 5 minutes.
- Remove from heat and mix with noodles. Transfer the mixture to a baking dish.
- In a small bowl, mix ricotta, parmesan, egg, and parsley. Spoon over the casserole.
- Bake 35-45 minutes until golden brown.

33 Salmon Keto Cutlets

Ingredients

- 450 g canned salmon
- ½ cup almond flour
- ¼ cup shallots, finely chopped

- 2 tbsp parsley, finely chopped
- 1 tbsp dried chopped onions
- 2 large eggs
- Zest of 1 lemon
- 1 clove garlic, finely chopped
- ½ tsp salt
- ½ tsp ground white pepper
- 3 tbsp olive oil

Cooking

- Put all the ingredients except the oil in a large bowl and mix well.
- Form 8 identical cutlets.
- Place a large non-stick pan over medium heat. Add half the butter.
- Fry salmon cutlets in portions, adding more oil as needed, for 2-3 minutes on each side.
- Serve the cutlets warm or cold with lemon wedges and low carbohydrate mayonnaise.

34 Brussels sprouts with maple syrup

Ingredients

- 2 tbsp olive oil

- 453.59 g Brussels sprouts, halved
- ½ tsp salt
- A pinch of ground black pepper
- 2 tbsp butter
- ½ cup pecans
- 2 tbsp sugarless maple syrup

Cooking

- Place a large non-stick pan over high heat and add olive oil.
- Put halves of cabbage in a pan with the cut side down, and sprinkle with salt and pepper.
- Fry for 3-4 minutes until brown and crispy, then turn over.
- Reduce heat to medium and add butter. Cook another 3 minutes.
- Add the pecans and mix.
- Once the cabbage is soft, add maple syrup without sugar. Throw the cabbage in a pan, and remove from heat.

35 Baked Cauliflower

Ingredients

- 1 medium cauliflower
- 113 g of salted butter

- ⅓ cup finely grated parmesan
- 3 tbsp Dijon mustard
- 2 minced garlic cloves
- Zest of 1 lemon
- ½ tsp salt
- ½ tsp ground pepper
- 28 g fresh Parmesan
- 1 tbsp finely chopped parsley

Cooking

- Preheat the oven to 190 degrees.
- Put the cauliflower in a small baking dish (I used a 9-inch).
- Put the remaining ingredients in a small saucepan, except for fresh parmesan and parsley, and put on low heat until they melt. Whip together.
- Lubricate cauliflower ⅓ of the oil mixture.
- Bake for 20 minutes, then remove from the oven and pour another quarter of the oil mixture.
- Bake for another 20 minutes and pour over the remaining oil mixture.
- Cook for another 20-30 minutes until the core is soft (check by inserting a small knife).
- Put on a plate, sprinkle a drop of oil from the mold, grate fresh parmesan and sprinkle with parsley.

36 Mushroom Risotto with Mushrooms

Recipe

- 2 tbsp olive oil
- 2 minced garlic cloves
- 1 small onion, finely diced
- 1 tsp salt
- ½ tsp ground white pepper
- 200 g chopped mushrooms
- ¼ cup chopped oregano leaves
- 255 g "rice" of cauliflower
- ¼ cup vegetable broth
- 2 tbsp butter
- ⅓ cup grated parmesan

Cooking

- Place a large non-stick pan over high heat.
- Add oil, garlic, onions, salt, and pepper, and sauté for 5-7 minutes until the onions become clear.
- Add mushrooms and oregano, and cook for 5 minutes.
- Add cauliflower rice and vegetable broth, then reduce heat to medium. Cook the risotto, stirring frequently, for 10-15 minutes, until the cauliflower is soft.
- Remove from heat, and mix with butter and parmesan.

- Try and add more seasoning if you want.

37 Low Carb Green Bean Casserole

Recipe

- 2 tbsp butter
- 1 small chopped onion
- 2 minced garlic cloves
- 226.8 g chopped mushrooms
- ½ tsp salt
- ½ tsp ground pepper
- ½ cup chicken stock
- ½ cup of fat cream
- ½ tsp xanthan gum
- 453.59 g green beans (with cut ends)
- 56.7 g crushed cracklings

Cooking

- Preheat the oven to 190 degrees.
- Add oil, onion, and garlic to a non-stick pan over high heat. Fry until onion is clear.
- Add mushrooms, salt, and pepper. Cook for 7 minutes until the mushrooms are tender.

- Add chicken stock and cream, and bring to a boil. Sprinkle with xanthan gum, mix and cook for 5 minutes.
- Add the string beans to the creamy mixture and pour it into the baking dish.
- Cover with foil and bake for 20 minutes.
- Remove the foil, sprinkle with greaves and bake for another 10-15 minutes.

38 French Zucchini (Gratin)

Recipe

- 2 tbsp butter or ghee ghee
- 2 garlic cloves, chopped
- 3 tbsp chopped fresh onions
- 125 g almond milk or heavy cream
- 226 g grated cheddar cheese
- 2 medium sliced zucchini

Cooking

- Melt the butter in a skillet over medium heat. Then add the garlic and onions, and cook until they are browned and fragrant.
- Add almond milk (or cream) and cook until it boils. Slowly add half the grated cheese and mix until it melts.
- Add chopped zucchini and mix well, covering the vegetables with the sauce. Cook another 5 minutes.
- Sprinkle the remaining cheese on top. Then bake in the oven at 204 ° C until the top is browned (about 20 minutes).

39 Avocado Low Carb Burger

Recipe

- 1 avocado
- 1 leaf lettuce
- 2 slices of prosciutto or any ham
- 1 slice of tomato
- 1 egg
- ½ tbsp olive oil for frying

For the sauce:

- 1 tbsp low carb mayonnaise
- ¼ tsp low carb hot sauce
- ¼ tsp mustard
- ¼ tsp Italian seasoning
- ½ tsp sesame seeds (optional

Cooking

- In a small bowl, combine keto-friendly mayonnaise, mustard, hot sauce, and Italian seasoning.
- Heat 1/2 tablespoon of olive oil in a pan and cook an egg. The yolk must be fluid.
- Cut the avocado in half, remove the peel and bone. Cut the narrowest part of the avocado so that the fruit can stand on a plate.
- Fill the hole in one half of the avocado with the prepared sauce.
- Top with lettuce, prosciutto strips, a slice of tomato and a fried egg.
- Cover with the other half of the avocado and sprinkle with sesame seeds (optional).

40 Italian sausages in a slow cooker with pepper

Recipe

- 283.5 g low-carb Italian sausages
- 1/2 chopped bell pepper
- 242 g canned tomatoes
- 1/2 chopped onion
- 1 clove of garlic
- 1 tsp Italian seasoning
- 1/2 tsp chopped red pepper
- 1/2 tsp sea salt
- 1/4 tsp black pepper
- 100 g grated Parmesan cheese

Cooking

- Arrange in a slow cooker: Italian sausages, bell peppers, onions, canned tomatoes, and minced garlic. Sprinkle with Italian seasoning, red pepper, sea salt, and pepper. Cook at low temperature for 6-8 hours.
- After cooking, put on plates and sprinkle with grated cheese.
- Serve with leafy greens, steamed broccoli or cauliflower rice.

41 Low carb goulash

Recipe

- 228 g shirataki noodles
- 0.5 tsp onion powder
- 2 minced garlic cloves
- 455 beef sausages or sausages
- 412 g diced tomatoes
- 25.25 g minced celery
- 1 pack of stevia
- 1 tsp salt
- 1 tsp chili powder

Cooking

- Drain the shirataki noodles, soak in water for 5 minutes, drain again, then fry in a dry pan, stirring constantly, until it starts to stick.
- Fry chopped sausage/sausages with onion powder and garlic until brown.
- Drain the fat as needed.
- Add the remaining ingredients.
- Stew for about 20 minutes, stirring often.

- Dinner recipes

42 Cauliflower and Pumpkin Casserole

Ingredients

- 2 tbsp. olive oil
- 1/4 medium yellow onion, minced
- 6 cups chopped forage kale into small pieces (about 140 g)
- 1 little clove garlic, minced
- Salt and freshly ground black pepper
- 1/2 cup low sodium chicken broth
- 2 cups of 1.5 cm diced pumpkin (about 230 g)
- 2 cups of 1.5 cm diced zucchini (about 230 g)
- 2 tbsp. mayonnaise
- 3 cups frozen, thawed brown rice
- 1 cup grated Swiss cheese
- 1/3 cup grated Parmesan
- 1 cup panko flour
- 1 large beaten egg
- Cooking spray

Preparation

4. Preheat oven to 200 ° C. Heats the oil in a large nonstick skillet over medium heat. Add onions and cook,

occasionally stirring, until browned and tender (about 5 minutes). Add the cabbage, garlic, and 1/2 teaspoon salt and 1/2 teaspoon pepper and cook until the cabbage is light (about 2 minutes).

5. Add the stock and continue to cook until the cabbage withers, and most of the stock evaporates (about 5 minutes). Add squash, zucchini, and 1/2 teaspoon salt and mix well. Continue cooking until the pumpkin begins to soften (about 8 minutes). Remove from heat and add mayonnaise.
6. In a bowl, combine cooked vegetables, brown rice, cheese, 1/2 cup flour, and large egg and mix well. Spray a 2-liter casserole with cooking spray. Spread the mixture across the bottom of the pan and cover with the remaining flour, 1/4 teaspoon salt and a few pinches of pepper. Bake until the squash and zucchini are tender and the top golden and crispy (about 35 minutes). Serve hot.

Advance Preparation Tip: Freeze the casserole for up to 2 weeks. Cover with aluminum foil and heat at 180 ° C until warm (35 to 45 minutes).

43 Thai beef salad Tears of the Tiger

Ingredients

- 800 g of beef tenderloin
- For the marinade :
- 2 tablespoons of soy sauce
- 1 tablespoon soup of honey
- 1 pinch of the pepper mill
- For the sauce :
- 1 small bunch of fresh coriander
- 1 small bouquet of mint
- 3 tablespoons soup of fish sauce
- lemon green
- 1 clove of garlic
- tablespoons soup of sugar palm (or brown sugar)
- 1 bird pepper or ten drops of Tabasco
- 1 small glass of raw Thai rice to make grilled rice powder
- 200 g of arugula or young shoots of salad

Preparation

- Cut the beef tenderloin into strips and put it in a container. Sprinkle with 2 tablespoons soy sauce, 1 tablespoon honey, and pepper. Although soak thoroughly and let marinate 1 hour at room temperature.
- Meanwhile, prepare the roasted rice powder. Pour a glass of Thai rice into an anti-adhesive pan. Dry color the rice, constantly stirring to avoid burning. When it has a lovely color, get rid of it on a plate and let it cool.

- When it has cooled, reduce it to powder by mixing it with the robot.
- Wash and finely chop mint and coriander. Put in a container and add lime juice, chopped garlic clove, 3 tablespoons Nuoc mam, 3 tablespoons brown sugar, 3 tablespoons water, 1 tablespoon sauce soy, and a dozen drops of Tabasco. Mix well and let stand the time that the sugar melts and the flavors mix.
- Place a bed of salad on a dish. Cook the beef strips put them on the salad. Sprinkle with the spoonful of sauce and roasted rice powder. To be served as is or with a Thai cooked white rice scented.

44 Stuffed apples with shrimp

Ingredients

- 6 medium apples
- 1 lemon juice
- 2 tablespoons butter

Filling:

- 300 gr of shrimp
- 1 onion minced
- ½ cup chopped parsley

- 2 tbsp flour
- 1 can of cream/cream
- 100 gr of curd
- 1 tablespoon butter
- 1 tbsp pepper sauce
- Salt to taste

Preparation

- Cut a cap from each apple, remove the seeds a little from the pulp on the sides, and put the pulp in the bottom, but leaving a cavity.
- Pass a little lemon and some butter on the apples, bake them in the oven. Remove from oven, let cool and bring to freeze.
- Prepare the shrimp sauce in a pan by mixing the butter with the flour, onion, parsley, and pepper sauce.
- Then add the prawn shrimp to the sauce. When boiling, mix the cream cheese and sour cream.
- Stuff each apple. Serve hot or cold, as you prefer.

45 A Quick Recipe of Grilled Chicken Salad with Oranges

Ingredients:

- 75 ml (1/3 cup) orange juice
- 30 ml (2 tablespoons) lemon juice
- 45 ml (3 tablespoons) of extra virgin olive oil
- 15 ml (1 tablespoon) Dijon mustard
- 2 cloves of garlic, chopped
- 1 ml (1/4 teaspoon) salt, or as you like
- Freshly ground pepper to your taste
- 1 lb. (450 g) skinless chicken breast, trimmed
- 25 g (1/4 cup) pistachio or flaked almonds, toasted
- 600 g (8c / 5 oz) of mesclun, rinsed and dried
- 75 g (1/2 cup) minced red onion
- 2 medium oranges, peeled, quartered and sliced

Preparation:

- Place the orange juice, lemon juice, oil, mustard, garlic, salt, and pepper in a small bowl or jar with an airtight lid;

whip or shake to mix. Reserve 75 milliliters (1/3 cup) of this salad vinaigrette and 45 milliliters (three tablespoons) for basting.

- Place the rest of the vinaigrette in a shallow glass dish or resealable plastic bag. Add the chicken and turn it over to coat. Cover or close and marinate in the refrigerator for at least 20 minutes or up to two hours.
- Preheat the barbecue over medium heat. Lightly oil the grill by rubbing it with a crumpled paper towel soaked in oil (use the tongs to hold the paper towel). Remove the chicken from the marinade and discard the marinade. Grill the chicken 10 to 15 centimeters (four to six inches) from the heat source, basting the cooked sides with the basting vinaigrette, until it is no longer pink in the center, and Instant-read thermometer inserted in the thickest part records 75 ° C (170 ° F), four to six minutes on each side. Transfer the chicken to a cutting board and let it rest for five minutes.
- Meanwhile, grill almonds (or pistachios) in a small, dry pan on medium-low heat, stirring constantly, until lightly browned, about two to three minutes. Transfer them to a bowl and let them cool.
- Place the salad and onion mixture in a large bowl. Mix with the vinaigrette reserved for the salad. Divide the salad into four plates. Slice chicken and spread on salads. Sprinkle

orange slices on top and sprinkle with pistachios (or almonds).

46 Red Curry with Vegetable

Ingredients

- 600 g sweet potatoes
- 200 g canned chickpeas
- 2 leek whites
- 2 tomatoes
- 100 g of spinach shoots
- 40 cl of coconut milk
- 1 jar of Greek yogurt
- 1 lime
- 3 cm fresh ginger
- 1 small bunch of coriander
- 1/2 red onion
- 2 cloves garlic
- 4 tbsp. red curry paste
- salt

Preparation

- Peel the sweet potatoes and cut them into pieces. Clean the leek whites and cut them into slices. Peel and seed the tomatoes.
- Mix the Greek yogurt with a drizzle of lime juice, chopped onion, salt, and half of the coriander leaves.
- In a frying pan, heat 15 cl of coconut milk until it reduces and forms a multitude of small bubbles. Brown curry paste with chopped ginger and garlic.
- Add vegetables, drained chickpeas, remaining coconut milk, and salt. Cook for 20 min covered, then 5 min without lid for the sauce to thicken.
- When serving, add spinach sprouts and remaining coriander. Serve with the yogurt sauce.

47 Baked Turkey Breast with Cranberry Sauce

Ingredients

- 2 kilos of whole turkey breast
- 1 tablespoon olive oil
- 1/4 cup onion
- 2 cloves of garlic
- thyme
- poultry seasonings

- you saved
- coarse-grained salt
- 2 butter spoons
- 1/4 cup minced echallot
- 1/4 cup chopped onion
- 1 clove garlic
- 2 tablespoons flour
- 1 1/2 cups of blueberries
- 2 cups apple cider
- 2 tablespoons maple honey
- peppers

Preparation

7. Grind in the blender ¼ cup onion, 2 garlic with herbs. Add 1 tablespoon of oil and spread the breast with this.
8. Put in the baking tray, add a cup of citron and bake at 350 Fahrenheit (180 ° C) to have a thermometer record 165 Fahrenheit (75 ° C) inside, about an hour, add ½ cup of water if necessary.
9. Bring the citron to a boil, add the blueberries, and leave a few minutes. In the butter (2 tablespoons), acitronar the onion (1/4 cup), echallot, and garlic (1 clove).
10. Add the flour to the onion and echallot and leave a few minutes. Add the citron, cranberries, and honey and leave on low heat. Season with salt and pepper, let the

blueberries are soft, go to the processor, and if you want to strain.

11. Return to the fire and let it thicken slightly.
12. Slice the thin turkey breast and serve with the blueberry sauce.

48 Low Carb Green Bean Casserole

Recipe

- 2 tbsp butter
- 1 small chopped onion
- 2 minced garlic cloves
- 226.8 g chopped mushrooms
- ½ tsp salt
- ½ tsp ground pepper
- ½ cup chicken stock
- ½ cup of fat cream
- ½ tsp xanthan gum
- 453.59 g green beans (with cut ends)
- 56.7 g crushed cracklings

Cooking

- Preheat the oven to 190 degrees.
- Add oil, onion, and garlic to a non-stick pan over high heat. Fry until onion is clear.
- Add mushrooms, salt, and pepper. Cook for 7 minutes until the mushrooms are tender.
- Add chicken stock and cream, and bring to a boil. Sprinkle with xanthan gum, mix and cook for 5 minutes.
- Add the string beans to the creamy mixture and pour it into the baking dish.
- Cover with foil and bake for 20 minutes.
- Remove the foil, sprinkle with greaves and bake for another 10-15 minutes.

49 French Zucchini (Gratin)

Recipe

- 2 tbsp butter or ghee ghee
- 2 garlic cloves, chopped
- 3 tbsp chopped fresh onions
- 125 g almond milk or heavy cream
- 226 g grated cheddar cheese
- 2 medium sliced zucchini

Cooking

- Melt the butter in a skillet over medium heat. Then add the garlic and onions, and cook until they are browned and fragrant.
- Add almond milk (or cream) and cook until it boils. Slowly add half the grated cheese and mix until it melts.
- Add chopped zucchini and mix well, covering the vegetables with the sauce. Cook another 5 minutes.
- Sprinkle the remaining cheese on top. Then bake in the oven at 204 ° C until the top is browned (about 20 minutes).

50 Avocado Low Carb Burger

Recipe

- 1 avocado
- 1 leaf lettuce
- 2 slices of prosciutto or any ham
- 1 slice of tomato
- 1 egg
- ½ tbsp olive oil for frying

For the sauce:

- 1 tbsp low carb mayonnaise
- ¼ tsp low carb hot sauce

- ¼ tsp mustard
- ¼ tsp Italian seasoning
- ½ tsp sesame seeds (optional

Cooking

- In a small bowl, combine keto-friendly mayonnaise, mustard, hot sauce, and Italian seasoning.
- Heat 1/2 tablespoon of olive oil in a pan and cook an egg. The yolk must be fluid.
- Cut the avocado in half, remove the peel and bone. Cut the narrowest part of the avocado so that the fruit can stand on a plate.
- Fill the hole in one half of the avocado with the prepared sauce.
- Top with lettuce, prosciutto strips, a slice of tomato and a fried egg.
- Cover with the other half of the avocado and sprinkle with sesame seeds (optional).

51 Italian sausages in a slow cooker with pepper

Recipe

- 283.5 g low-carb Italian sausages
- 1/2 chopped bell pepper
- 242 g canned tomatoes
- 1/2 chopped onion
- 1 clove of garlic
- 1 tsp Italian seasoning
- 1/2 tsp chopped red pepper
- 1/2 tsp sea salt
- 1/4 tsp black pepper
- 100 g grated Parmesan cheese

Cooking

- Arrange in a slow cooker: Italian sausages, bell peppers, onions, canned tomatoes, and minced garlic. Sprinkle with Italian seasoning, red pepper, sea salt, and pepper. Cook at low temperature for 6-8 hours.
- After cooking, put on plates and sprinkle with grated cheese.
- Serve with leafy greens, steamed broccoli or cauliflower rice.

52 Low carb goulash

Recipe

- 228 g shirataki noodles
- 0.5 tsp onion powder
- 2 minced garlic cloves
- 455 beef sausages or sausages
- 412 g diced tomatoes
- 25.25 g minced celery
- 1 pack of stevia
- 1 tsp salt
- 1 tsp chili powder

Cooking

- Drain the shirataki noodles, soak in water for 5 minutes, drain again, then fry in a dry pan, stirring constantly, until it starts to stick.
- Fry chopped sausage/sausages with onion powder and garlic until brown.
- Drain the fat as needed.
- Add the remaining ingredients.
- Stew for about 20 minutes, stirring often.

53 Low carb egg noodles

Ingredient

- 3 egg yolks
- 113.4 g soft cream cheese
- 0.13 tsp garlic powder fresh grated Parmesan cheese (about 1/3 cup plus 2 tablespoons)
- 37.33 g of freshly grated mozzarella cheese (about 1/3 cup plus 2 tablespoons)
- 0.13 tsp dried basil
- 0.13 tsp dried marjoram
- 0.13 tsp dried tarragon
- 0.13 tsp ground oregano
- 0.13 tsp ground black pepper

Cooking

- Beat egg yolks and cream cheese together. Add the parmesan and mozzarella, and continue whisking. Sprinkle with spices and beat well again.
- Put a baking sheet on parchment, and evenly distribute the cheese-egg mixture on it. Smooth with a spatula or the back of a spoon.

- Place the pan in the preheated oven to 246 ° C and reduce the temperature to 176 ° C.
- Bake 5 to 8 minutes. If small bubbles begin to appear, reduce the temperature to 148 ° C and continue to bake for 2-3 minutes until cooked.
- Let cool at room temperature for 10 to 15 minutes. Slice with a regular pizza knife or knife.

54 Baked ratatouille

Recipe

- 1 green zucchini
- 1 yellow zucchini
- 3 large tomatoes
- 1 eggplant
- 3 tbsp olive oil
- 1 tsp garlic powder
- 1/4 cup fresh basil
- 1 tsp salt
- 1 tsp black pepper
- 1 tsp oregano
- 1 cup low-carb tomato sauce
- Not necessary:

- 3 tbsp pesto
- 1/4 cup crumbled feta cheese

Cooking

- Thinly chop the vegetables.
- In a bowl, combine oil, garlic powder, oregano, salt, and black pepper.
- Put the chopped vegetables in a bowl of butter and seasonings, and mix.
- Put the tomato sauce on the bottom of the baking dish/dish.
- Lay the slices of vegetables on top, vertically in a circle.
- Place fresh basil between the slices.
- Cover the dish with foil and bake at a temperature of 170 degrees for 40 minutes.
- Remove the foil and make sure the vegetables are tender. Bake another 20 minutes without a lid.

55 Avocado roll with a vegetable salad

Recipe

- 55 g soft cream cheese
- 4 eggs, protein separated from yolks
- 150 g full whipped cream
- 200 g grated cheddar cheese
- 1/2 tsp salt
- 1/2 tsp black pepper
- 50 g grated Parmesan cheese

Filling

- Mashed 1 avocado
- 1 chopped cucumber
- 6 chopped cherry tomatoes
- 1/2 cup lettuce

Cooking

- Preheat the oven to 200 degrees.
- Beat cream cheese and egg yolk together.
- Add cream and mix.
- Add grated cheddar cheese and seasonings.
- In another bowl, beat the egg whites until foamy.
- Gently add the egg whites to the creamy mixture.

- Pour into a rectangular baking sheet with parchment.
- Sprinkle with half the cheese on top and bake for 12-15 minutes.
- Place a piece of parchment paper on the kitchen surface and sprinkle with the remaining parmesan cheese.
- Remove the roll from the oven, place it face down on parmesan-coated paper and let cool. Remove the top paper.
- Spread mashed avocado on a roll.
- Then sprinkle slices of cucumber, tomato, and lettuce.

Roll up the roll, starting at one of the long edges, using the paper at the

56 Tomato cream of red lentils

Components

- ¾ cup dry red lentils
- 1-2 canned tomatoes pelati (in season 2-4 cups of sliced fresh)
- 1 white onion
- 1 clove of garlic
- 1 large carrot
- 1 tablespoon oil rapeseed

- 1-2 tablespoons of juice of a lemon
- 1 -2 teaspoon cumin (cumin)
- 1 teaspoon smoked pepper (preferably acute)
- 1 teaspoon savory or lovage
- teaspoon thyme
- decoction vegetable or water
- salt, pepper
- to serve: buckwheat, parsley, coriander

Process

- In a thick-bottomed pot or deep saucepan, heat the oil and fry the finely chopped onion, then add garlic.
- Then add the diced carrot and the washed lentils and pour the vegetable stock so that it fully covers all ingredients to a height of 2-3 cm. Cook until carrots and lentils are soft.
- When the vegetables soften, add canned tomatoes and spices. Boil for another 10-15 minutes, then blend with a hand blender, add lemon juice and season to taste. Serve with buckwheat and fresh herbs.

57 Simple miso soup - for a cold!

Ingredients

- 500 ml of water or vegan dashi broth
- 2 - 3 tablespoons light miso paste
- half a bunch of onions spring onions
- 100 grams of natural tofu or more
- 1 sheet of nori
- Pak Choy algae , any green leafy vegetable, even our good kale
- soy sauce (optional)

Process

- Boil water in a medium saucepan and add chopped burrow algae into small rectangles. Boil and keep on very low or even off the fire. Add miso paste and mix thoroughly. You can mix it in a small amount of water and only then add to the entire saucepan - there will be no lumps.
- Dice the tofu, chop the spring onions and green park Choy / kale leaves and add them to the hot soup. Instead of salt (although the paste itself is quite salty already), add soy sauce to the soup - if you feel the need.
- Hold the stove for a while, and it's ready! Serve in small bowls with extra spring onions

58 Warming cream of baked vegetables

Ingredients

- 3 smaller carrots
- half of the medium celery root
- 1 sweet potato
- 1 medium plain potato
- 1 medium white onion
- 4 cloves of garlic
- 1 teaspoon grated fresh ginger
- 3 teaspoons tomato paste
- 2 tablespoons olive oil
- ½ liter - 1-liter vegetable broth fungal or
- 1 teaspoon pepper smoked, e.g., the
- 1 teaspoon of hot pepper, for example. the
- half teaspoon cumin
- salt and pepper
- to give: toasts, cream Sunflower

Process

- Scrub the sweet potato, carrot, potato, and celery thoroughly, peel only the celery. Cut them all into 2 cm cubes and put them in a wide bowl. Add tomato paste and rub all the vegetables with it, it's best done with your hands.
- Heat the oven to 190 degrees, line the baking tray with baking paper and spread the vegetables on it along with

the peeled garlic. Bake until all the vegetables are soft and remove the garlic earlier, after about 15 minutes, so that it does not burn and is not bitter.

- In the meantime, fry the chopped onion in the frying pan with olive oil until it is vitrified. Add the grated ginger now and choke everything for a moment, stirring vigorously.
- Put the roasted vegetables into a pot or a blender and add onion and ginger. Mix at low speed, adding a little broth until you get the consistency you want. Add spices and season with salt and pepper.
- Serve with warm croutons, a blend of sunflower cream, and your favorite sprouts.

59 Watermelon gazpacho in a jar

Ingredients

- 1kg of ripe, aromatic tomatoes (I use a buffalo heart)
- half a red pepper +
- half a small chili pepper
- 3 ground cucumbers
- 1 onion
- 1 clove of garlic (optional)
- 2 cups cubed watermelon

- juice of 1 lemon
- a handful of leaves basil
- a handful of mint leaves
- 1 - 2 tablespoons olive oil
- salt, pepper

Process

- Tomato peel slightly cut in several places, then transfer the tomatoes to a deep pot and pour boiling water, let stand for a few minutes. Drain the water and peel the tomatoes from the skin, but this is not a necessary stage if the skin does not bother you.
- Peeled tomatoes in half and put in a blender cup or larger bowl. Add chopped onion, garlic, diced peppers, cucumbers, chili peppers, and lemon juice. Also, add basil and mint leaves. All mix well in a blender or using a hand blender, finally adding olive oil.
- Then add chopped pieces of watermelon and mix only for a moment, so that the remaining watermelon particles can be felt. Season with salt and pepper to taste.
- Serve well chilled with diced paprika, lemon juice, stale bread, and a large dose of fresh, chopped basil.

60 Mango soup with cider and chili

Ingredients

- 3 large pieces of ripe, soft mango
- approx. 150 ml of cider or mineral water
- 1 medium chili pepper
- 3 pinches of cardamom
- 1 tablespoon of coconut milk or soy cream (optional, but I recommend)
- fresh mint leaves

Process

- Peel the mango by removing pieces from the stone and then separating the flesh from the skin. Transfer them to a hand blender, cup blender, or one with "S" knives.
- Add a little water or cider; mix everything into a smooth cream, gradually adding the liquid until you get the consistency you want. Then add a little coconut milk or vegan cream.
- Pour the cooler into an airtight container or jar and cool to a low temperature, before serving you can even keep it in the freezer for a while.
- Serve the cooler in a bowl and add chopped chili on top of the liquid (remember to wash your hands and all tools that have come into contact with the chili) and fresh mint. Stir everything before eating.

61 Peanut sweet potato ginger cream

Ingredients

- 1 larger sweet potato (about 400 - 500g)
- 1 leek (white and light green part)
- 1 carrot
- 1 clove of garlic a
- bit of olive oil
- 2 - 3 tablespoons of peanut butter (the best will be without salt)
- 2cm fresh ginger, grated on a grater
- 1.5l vegetable broth a
- few pinches of pepper (hot or fresh)
- salt, pepper

Process

- Peel the garlic and chop it with the leek, then fry in a large pot on the hot oil until the leek is soft.
- Add diced sweet potato and carrot (I do not peel, I scrub properly). Add a little salt and pepper, stew for a few minutes.
- Pour over the vegetable broth and cook on medium heat until sweet potato and carrot are soft.

- When the vegetables are ready, add the ginger and mix it into a smooth cream.
- Then add the peanut butter before mixing it in a small bowl with a little cream - so that the butter mixes well. Season to taste with salt and pepper and paprika. Eat with croutons (e.g., baked) tofu, sprouts, or good bread, tasty!

62 Pumpkin spice syrup

Ingredients

- ¾ cup thick coconut milk
- 1 cup pumpkin purée
- ¾ cup brown sugar
- ½ cup soy or almond milk 1 mig
- teaspoon ground cinnamon
- ½ teaspoon ground vanilla (or 1 teaspoon vanilla extract)
- 1 teaspoon anise grains
- pinch of salt

Process

- Heat coconut milk in a saucepan, add sugar, pumpkin puree (baked and mixed pumpkin), and all spices. If you use very thick mashed potatoes, add some soy milk to get a smooth consistency. 2. Hold it for several minutes on low heat until the sugar dissolves and the liquid thickens a Little. Season again to taste, without forgetting the salt, which conquers all other spices by itself. 3. Pour the syrup through a sieve into a medium bottle, and when it cools down, close it tightly. You can store it in the fridge for several weeks.

63 Matcha vegan cheesecake

Ingredients

- 2-3 teaspoons matcha tea
- ½ cup maple syrup (or agave)
- ¼ cup of coconut oil
- juice from 1 lemon a
- bit of vanilla extract a
- pinch of salt a
- few spoons of pistachios

Process

- Prepare your favorite cheesecake bottom and transfer it to a sheet covered with cling film.
- Soak cashews in water - preferably all night or 2-3 hours in boiling water. Transfer them to a blender together with syrup, oil, extract, and salt. Mix everything to a smooth

mass, the longer - the consistency will be creamier. At the end of mixing, add lemon juice, controlling the sour taste of the mass - I like it when the mass is quite acidic, but you can overdo it.

- Put just over half the weight into the previously prepared mold on the bottom. Add the matcha tea gradually to the remaining mass, mixing all the time until all the lumps disappear. Every now and then, check if the tea is already palatable so as not to overdose it - the mass may come out too bitter.
- Tap the cheesecake tray on the kitchen counter to get rid of air from the mass. Sprinkle the top of the cheesecake with chopped pistachios and transfer to the freezer. The cheesecake will be ready after a few hours, and before eating, pull it out about 30 minutes before serving.

➢ Desserts And Sweets

64 Oatmeal and berry muffins

INGREDIENTS

- 1 cup (250 mL) non-blanched all-purpose flour
- ½ cup (125 mL) quick-cooking oatmeal 1/2 cup
- (160 mL) stuffed brown sugar
- 1/2 tbsp (1/2 cup) tea) baking soda

- 2 eggs
- 125 ml (1/2 cup) applesauce
- 60 ml (1/4 cup)
- orange canola oil 1, grated rind only
- 1 lemon, grated rind
- 15 ml (1 tbsp) lemon juice
- 180 ml (3/4 cup) fresh raspberries (see note)
- 180 ml (3/4 cup) fresh or blueberries (or blackberries)

PREPARATION

1. Put the grill at the center of the oven. Preheat oven to 180 ° C (350 ° F). Line 12 muffin cups with paper or silicone trays.
2. In a bowl, combine flour, oatmeal, brown sugar, and baking soda. Book.
3. In a big bowl, whisk together eggs, applesauce, oil, citrus zest, and lemon juice. Add the dry ingredients to the wooden spoon. Add the berries and mix gently.
4. Spread the mixture in the boxes. Sprinkle top with pistachio muffins. Bake for 20 to 22 minutes or until a toothpick inserted in the center of a muffin comes out clean. Let cool.

65 Crunchy Blueberry and Apples

INGREDIENTS

Crunchy

- 1 cup (1¼ cup) quick-cooking oatmeal
- ¼ cup (60 mL) brown sugar
- ¼ cup (60 mL) unbleached all-purpose flour
- 90 ml (6 tablespoons) melted margarine

Garnish

- 125 ml (½ cup) brown sugar
- 20 ml (4 teaspoons) cornstarch
- 1 liter (4 cups) fresh or frozen blueberries (not thawed)
- 500 ml (2 cups) grated apples
- 1 Tbsp.
- (15 mL) melted margarine 15 mL (1 tablespoon) lemon juice

PREPARATION

1. Put the grill at the center of the oven. Preheat oven to 180 ° C (350 ° F).
2. In a bowl, mix dry ingredients. Add the margarine and mix until the mixture is just moistened. Book.

3. In a 20-cm (8-inch) square baking pan, combine brown sugar and cornstarch. Add the fruits, margarine, lemon juice, and mix well. Cover with crisp and bake between 55 minutes and 1 hour, or until the crisp is golden brown. Serve warm or cold.

66 Fresh Cranberry Pie

INGREDIENTS

- 1 ½ cup crumbled Graham crackers
- ¼ cup salt-free chopped pecans
- 1 ¾ cup Splenda Sweetener
- ½ cup non-hydrogenated salt-free margarine
- 1 ½ cup freshly picked cranberries
- 2 egg whites
- 1 tbsp. thawed apple juice concentrate
- 1 tbsp. vanilla extract

- 1 liter Cool Whip Whipped Topping, thawed

Cranberry Frosting:

- ¼ cup Splenda Sweetener
- ¼ cup caster sugar
- 1 Tbsp. cornstarch
- ¾ cup fresh cranberries
- ¾ cup of water

PREPARATION

1. Preheat oven to 375 ° F (190 ° C).
2. Mix crumbled crackers, pecans, and ¾ cup of Splenda. Add the margarine, mix well, and arrange on a hinged mold pressing on the bottom and the sides. Bake dough for 6 minutes or until slightly browned, let cool.
3. Mix the cranberries with 1 cup of Splenda. Let stand for 5 minutes. Add the egg whites, apple juice, and vanilla. Beat at low speed until foamy, and then beat at high speed for 5 to 8 minutes until mixture is firm.

4. Stir in the whipped topping in the cranberry mixture. Pour the mixture over the pre-cooked dough. Refrigerate at least 4 hours until the mixture is firm.
5. To make the icing, mix the sugar, Splenda, and cornstarch in a saucepan. Stir in cranberries and water. Cook, stirring until bubbles appear. Continue cooking, occasionally stirring until cranberry skin comes off. Use the mixture at room temperature. Do not refrigerate: the sauce may crystallize and become opaque.
6. Remove the tart from the pan and arrange on a serving platter, using a spoon, coat with icing.

67 Low carb chocolate mousse

INGREDIENTS

- 300 ml whipping cream
- ½ tsp vanilla extract
- 2 egg yolks
- 1 pinch salt
- 100 g dark chocolate with a minimum of 80% cocoa solids

INSTRUCTIONS

- Break or cut the chocolate into small pieces. Melt in the microwave (at intervals of 20 seconds, stirring each time) or using a water bath. Reserve to cool to room temperature.
- Beat the cream until it is about to snow. Add the vanilla towards the end.
- Mix the egg yolks with the salt in a separate bowl.
- Add the melted chocolate to the yolks and mix until you have a uniform consistency dough.
- Add a couple of tablespoons of whipped cream to the chocolate mixture and stir to make it a little more liquid. Add the remaining cream and add it to the mixture.
- Divide the dough into ramequins or serving glasses. Put in the refrigerator and let cool for at least 2 hours. Serve alone or with fresh berries.

68 Chocolate Keto Cake with Peanut Butter Cream

INGREDIENTS

- 225 ml (110 g) ground almonds
- 175 ml (125 g) erythritol
- 125 ml (50 g) cocoa powder
- 1½ tbsp (12 g) psyllium powder husks

- 1 tbsp baking powder
- ¼ tsp Salt
- 4 eggs
- 225 g (225 ml) cream cheese
- 110 g melted salted butter
- Peanut Butter Frosting
- 225 g salted butter
- 225 g (225 ml) cream cheese
- 125 ml unsalted and unsweetened peanut butter
- 60 ml (50 g) erythritol, powder
- 2 tsp vanilla extract
- Ornaments
- 10 cherries (optional)
- 125 ml whipping cream
- 1 tbsp (10 g) salted peanuts, chopped

INSTRUCTIONS

- Place the rack in the center of the oven and preheat to 180 ° C (350 ° F).
- Mix almond flour, sweetener, cocoa powder (filter to remove lumps), ground psyllium husk powder, baking powder, and salt in a medium bowl. Beat until well mixed. Reserve.
- Pour the eggs into a large bowl. Beat with the electric pastry mixer for a couple of minutes until they are fluffy.

Add cream cheese and melted butter. Continue beating until the mixture is smooth and homogeneous.

- Add the flour mixture in the bowl with the eggs and beat a couple of minutes until the cake dough is smooth.
- Grease two cake moulds 18 cm (7 inches), or do it one by one if you only have one mold. Pour half of the dough into each mold and distribute it evenly. Bake for 15-20 minutes or until a toothpick in the center comes out clean.
- Allow cooling for at least 10 minutes in the mold before passing it to a rack to cool. Wrap the layers with plastic wrap and place in the refrigerator; let cool completely, preferably overnight.

69 Low carb chocolate peanut squares

INGREDIENTS

- 100 g dark chocolate with a minimum of 70% cocoa solids
- 4 tbsp butter or coconut oil
- 1 pinch salt
- 60 ml of peanut butter
- ½ tsp vanilla extract
- 1 tsp powdered licorice or ground cardamom (green)
- 60 ml (35 g) chopped salted peanuts, for decoration

INSTRUCTIONS

- Melt the chocolate and butter or coconut oil in the microwave or in a water-bath pot. If you don't have a pot for a water bath, you can put a glass bowl on top of a pot with boiling water. Make sure the water does not reach the container. The chocolate will melt by the heat of the steam. Mix all other ingredients and pour the mixture into a small roasting pan lined with baking paper (no larger than 10 x 15 centimeters).
- Let cool for a while and cover with finely chopped peanuts or other creative toppings. Refrigerate.
- When the dough is ready, cut it into small squares with a sharp knife. Remember that all whims are small, not more than a square of 2.5 cm x 2.5 cm. Store in the refrigerator or freezer.

➢ Entries and Snacks

70 Eggplant and chickpea bites

INGREDIENTS

- 3 large aubergines cut in half (make a few cuts in the flesh with a knife) Spray
- oil
- 2 large cloves garlic, peeled and deglazed
- 2 tbsp. coriander powder
- 2 tbsp. cumin seeds
- 400 g canned chickpeas, rinsed and drained
- 2 Tbsp. chickpea flour
- Zest and juice of 1/2 lemon
- 1/2 lemon quartered for serving
- 3 tbsp. tablespoon of polenta

PREPARATION

- Heat the oven to 200°C (180°C rotating heat, gas level 6). Spray the eggplant halves generously with oil and place them on the meat side up on a baking sheet. Sprinkle with coriander and cumin seeds, and then place the cloves of garlic on the plate. Season and roast for 40 minutes until the flesh of eggplant is completely tender. Reserve and let cool a little.

- Scrape the flesh of the eggplant in a bowl with a spatula and throw the skins in the compost. Thoroughly scrape and make sure to incorporate spices and crushed roasted garlic. Add chickpeas, chickpea flour, zest, and lemon juice. Crush roughly and mix well, check to season. Do not worry if the mixture seems a bit soft - it will firm up in the fridge.
- Form about twenty pellets and place them on a baking sheet covered with parchment paper. Let stand in the fridge for at least 30 minutes.
- Preheat oven to 180°C (rotating heat 160°C, gas level 4). Remove the meatballs from the fridge and coat them by rolling them in the polenta. Place them back on the baking sheet and spray a little oil on each. Roast for 20 minutes until golden and crisp. Serve with lemon wedges. You can also serve these dumplings with a spicy yogurt dip with harissa, this delicious but spicy mashed paste of hot peppers and spices from the Maghreb.

71 Baba Ghanouj

INGREDIENTS

- 1 large aubergine, cut in half lengthwise
- 1 head of garlic, unpeeled
- 30 ml (2 tablespoons) of olive oil
- Lemon juice to taste

PREPARATION

- Put the grill at the center of the oven. Preheat the oven to 350 ° F. Line a baking sheet with parchment paper.
- Place the eggplant on the plate, skin side up. Roast until the meat is very tender and detaches easily from the skin, about 1 hour depending on the size of the eggplant. Let cool.
- Meanwhile, cut the tip of the garlic cloves. Place the garlic cloves in a square of aluminum foil. Fold the edges of the sheet and fold together to form a tightly wrapped foil. Roast with the eggplant until tender, about 20 minutes. Let cool. Purée the pods with a garlic press.
- With a spoon, scoop out the flesh of the eggplant and place it in the bowl of a food processor. Add the garlic puree, the oil, and the lemon juice. Stir until purée is smooth and pepper.
- Serve with mini pita bread.

72 Spicy crab dip

INGREDIENTS

- 1 can of 8 oz softened cream cheese
- 1 tbsp. to . finely chopped onions
- 1 tbsp. at . lemon juice
- 2 tbsp. at . Worcestershire sauce
- 1/8 tsp. at t. black
- pepper Cayenne pepper to taste
- 2 tbsp. to s. of milk or non-fortified rice drink
- 1 can of 6 oz of crabmeat

PREPARATION

- Preheat the oven to 375 ° F (190 ° C).
- Pour the cream cheese into a bowl. Add the onions, lemon juice, Worcestershire sauce, black pepper, and cayenne pepper. Mix well. Stir in the milk/rice drink. Add the crabmeat and mix until you obtain a homogeneous mixture.
- Pour the mixture into a baking dish. Cook without covering for 15 minutes or until bubbles appear. Serve hot with low-sodium crackers or triangle cut pita bread. OR
- Microwave until bubbles appear, about 4 minutes, stirring every 1 to 2 minutes.

73 Potatoes" of Parmesan cheese

Ingredients

- 75 g grated Parmesan cheese
- 1 tbsp (8 g) Chia seeds
- 2 tbsp (20 g) whole flaxseeds
- 2½ tbsp (20 g) pumpkin seeds

Instructions

- Preheat the oven to 180 ° C (350 ° F).
- Cover a baking sheet with baking paper.
- Mix the cheese and seeds in a bowl.
- With a spoon, put small piles of the mixture on the baking paper, leaving some space between them. Do not flatten the piles. Bake for 8 to 10 minutes checks frequently. "Potatoes" should take a light brown color, but not dark brown.
- Remove from the oven and let cool before removing the "potatoes" from the paper and serve them.

74 Chili cheese chicken with crispy and delicious cabbage salad

INGREDIENTS

Chili Cheese Chicken

- 400 grams of chicken
- 200 grams of tomatoes
- 100 grams of cream cheese
- 125 grams of cheddar
- 40 grams of jalapenos
- 60 grams of bacon

Crispy Cabbage Salad

- 0.5 pcs casserole
- 200 grams of Brussels sprouts
- grams of almonds
- 3 paragraph mandarins
- 1 tablespoon olive oil
- 1 teaspoon apple cider vinegar
- 0.5 tsp salt
- 0.25 teaspoon pepper
- 1 tablespoon lemon

PREPARATION

- Turn on the oven at 200 °. Cut tomatoes in half and place in the bottom of a dish. Put chicken fillets in the dish, place half of the cream cheese on each chicken fillet and sprinkle with cheddar. Spread jalapenos in the dish and bake it first for 25 minutes. Place bacon on a baking sheet with baking paper, and bake it for 10 minutes. Next, make the cabbage salad. When the chicken dish has been given 35 minutes, it should be done
- Put the Brussels sprouts and cumin in a food processor and blend it well and thoroughly. Make the dressing of juice from one mandarin, olive oil, apple cider vinegar, salt, pepper, and lemon juice. Put the cabbage in a dish and spread the dressing over. Chop almonds, cut the tangerine into slices and place it on the salad.
- Sprinkle the bacon over the chicken dish before serving, and serve it with the cabbage salad!

75 KETO pumpkin pie for Halloween, sweet and spicy

INGREDIENTS

Pie Bottom

- 110 grams of almond flour
- 50 grams of sucrine
- 0.5 tsp salt
- grams of protein powder 1 scoop
- 1 paragraph eggs
- 80 grams of butter
- 15 grams of fiber

The Filling

- 1 pcs Hokkaido
- 3 paragraph egg yolks
- 60 ml of coconut milk the fat, not the water
- 1 teaspoon vanilla powder
- 15 grams of protein powder
- 1 teaspoon cinnamon
- grams of sucrine
- 0.5 tsp cardamom Bla
- 0.5 tsp cloves

PREPARATION

- Preheat oven to 175 °. Start making the bottom as it needs to be baked!
- Mix all the dry ingredients in a bowl and add the wet ones. Stir it well and take over with your hands so you can shape it into a lump. Take a piece of baking paper and place the dough lump. Place a piece of baking paper on top and flatten the dough. Shape it to the size of a regular pie mold 24 cm in diameter. Use a rolling pin if necessary. Prick holes in the bottom and behind dough in the oven for 8-10 minutes. Be careful about giving it too much (we did it the first time)
- Then make the filling. Cut the meat off your Hokkaido (or the garbage off the meat!) And cook it in a saucepan for 15-20 minutes. Put it in a food processor and add all the other ingredients and blend it well.
- Pour the stuffing into the baked pie and bake again for approx. 25-30 minutes more until it looks golden and done. Eat when cool or cool down first. A dollop of whipped cream is great too!

CONCLUSION

Keto foods provide a high per calory amount of protein. This is important because the basal metabolic rate (the number of calories required daily for survival) is less for the aged, but they still need the same amount of nutrients as the younger.

A person 50+ will live on junk foods much harder than a teen or 20-something whose body is still resilient. This makes eating foods that are health-supporting and disease-fighting even more important for seniors. It can literally mean the difference between fully enjoying the golden years or wasting them in pain and agony.

Seniors therefore need to eat a more optimal diet by avoiding "empty calories" from sugars or anti-nutrient-rich foods, such as whole grains, and by increasing their amount of nutrient-rich fats and protein.

However, much of the food preferred by older people (or delivered in a hospital or clinical setting) appears to be heavily processed and very low in nutrients such as white pieces of bread, kinds of pasta, prunes, mashed potatoes, puddings etc.

In short, we're all getting older and death is imminent, of course. But the quality of life along the way is what we CAN manage to some degree. People are living longer today, but we get sicker also by adopting the majority's standard diet. The ketogenic diet can

help seniors improve their health, so they can actually thrive in the later years of their lives, rather than being ill or in pain.

CPSIA information can be obtained
at www.ICGtesting.com
Printed in the USA
LVHW060739081220
672143LV00041B/7